Maggie Jones is the author of fifteen books, both non-
fiction and fiction. She specializes in health issues,
writing regularly for national magazines and newspapers,
and has a particular interest in children's health.

YOUR CHILD SERIES

A series of books containing easy-to-follow, practical advice for the parents of children with a variety of illnesses or conditions.

Each book provides a clear overview of the situation, explaining essential information about the illness or condition and outlining the practical steps parents can take to help understand, support and care for their child, the rest of the family as well as themselves. Guiding parents through the conventional, the complementary and the alternative approaches which are available, these books cater for children of all ages, ranging from babies to teenagers, and enable the whole family to move forward in a positive way.

Titles in the *Your Child* series:

Your Child: *Allergies* by Brigid McConville with Dr Rajendra Sharma
Your Child: *Asthma* by Erika Harvey
Your Child: *Bullying* by Jenny Alexander
Your Child: *Diabetes* by Catherine Steven
Your Child: *Dyslexia* by Robin Temple
Your Child: *Eczema* by Maggie Jones
Your Child: *Epilepsy* by Fiona Marshall
Your Child: *Headaches & Migraine* by Maggie Jones

YOUR CHILD

Headaches & Migraine

Practical and Easy-to-Follow Advice

Maggie Jones

ELEMENT
Shaftesbury, Dorset • Boston, Massachusetts
Melbourne, Victoria

© Element Books Limited 1999
Text © Maggie Jones 1999

First published in the UK in 1999 by
Element Books Limited
Shaftesbury, Dorset SP7 8BP

Published in the USA in 1999 by
Element Books, Inc.
160 North Washington Street
Boston, MA 02114

Published in Australia in 1999 by
Element Books and distributed
by Penguin Australia Limited
487 Maroondah Highway, Ringwood,
Victoria 3134

Cover photograph © Pictor International
Cover design by Slatter-Anderson
Design by Roger Lightfoot
Typeset by Intype London Ltd
Printed and bound in Great Britain by
Creative Print and Design (Wales), Ebbw Vale

British Library Cataloguing in Publication
data available

Library of Congress Cataloging in Publication data available

ISBN 1 86204 397 3

Contents

Introduction

There is increasing evidence that more children and young people today are suffering from regular headaches and migraines. While almost everyone has had a headache and knows how it feels, not everyone understands what migraine is. It can sometimes be difficult to distinguish between recurrent headaches and migraine, but on the whole a migraine is a severe headache which may be accompanied by strange visual symptoms, nausea and vomiting. People can, generally put up with an occasional migraine, but migraines usually occur regularly, sometimes as often as once a week or once a fortnight. Unlike ordinary headaches, which usually stop when the person rests or takes painkillers, a migraine attack usually has to run its course, sometimes lasting as long as two or three days.

It is not commonly known that children as well as adults can suffer from migraine. An estimated one in nine children between the ages of 5 and 15 are affected. However, the line between the definition of 'migraine' and recurrent or frequent headaches is not clear, and if migraines and recurrent tension headaches are counted together, as many as one in five children may be affected.

It used to be thought that migraine is very uncommon under the age of five, but new research shows this is not so. Migraine in a very young child often presents simply as nausea, vomiting and general prostration, with the child sometimes crying in pain. Because a young child cannot explain its symptoms, the headache is often unrecognized and a 'tummy upset' or 'bilious attack' is usually diagnosed. Children find it difficult to be specific about symptoms or locate a source of pain. One young boy told his mother repeatedly that he had a tummy ache. When the mother took him to the doctor and the doctor started to examine his tummy, the child said, 'No, it's a tummy ache in my head'.

The incidence of migraine increases with age, becoming more common in adolescence and young adulthood, and levelling off around middle age. At least one in three adult sufferers say that their migraines started before the age of ten. In young children migraine is more common in boys, but many girls start to suffer from migraines when their periods start. In women, 60 per cent of migraines are connected with their menstrual cycle, with migraines being most common just before a period. Migraine in children seems to be more common when one or more parents has suffered from migraine, but it is not clear whether this is because the capacity is inherited, or because children 'learn' this way of dealing with stress. However, there is probably a genetic element predisposing people to this condition.

If you haven't suffered from migraine yourself, it can be difficult to understand what your child is feeling. While parents do obviously feel sympathy, repeated migraine attacks can be very inconvenient for the whole family, upsetting long-term plans, disrupting arrangements and tying you and your child to your home. Sometimes parents suspect that their child is using a 'headache' as a way of getting off school, or is exaggerating the symptoms because they wish to avoid doing something the parents want them to do, such as going to a piano lesson or visiting elderly relatives. Some children with less severe migraine want to carry on as usual and suppress their symptoms, while seeming bad tempered, low in energy and depressed.

In other cases, a child simply has a headache with no nausea or vomiting, and migraine may not be diagnosed at all. Indeed, the definition of migraine is not really at all clear. In 'classical' migraine, with an aura and visual disturbances, it is easy to diagnose. But 'common' migraine occurs far more frequently, and the symptoms may be the same as for recurrent tension headaches. Children – and adults – are not always completely prostrated with migraine. As one nine-year-old described it, 'It's like having a heavy head and feeling seasick at the same time'.

Doctors themselves are not always clear about the distinction between headaches and migraine. Any recurrent headache is likely to be similar to migraine and may have the same triggers and respond to the same treatment.

Migraine attacks can last for as little as two hours or as long as two or three days. In children, the vomiting can be so severe that there is a danger of dehydration and a very small number of children need to be admitted to hospital so that they can have intravenous fluids. Fortunately, most migraines are not this severe, though they are very unpleasant while they last.

As with adults, many children who suffer from migraine may experience an 'aura' before an attack. This can be a partial loss of vision, flashing lights and spots before the eyes, rather like those you get after looking at the sun or a camera flash. Children may rub their eyes, act as if confused, or say things like, 'Has the room gone dark?', 'There are snakes in front of my eyes', 'I can see spots'. Sometimes the child can hear things, has a strange taste in the mouth, feels dizzy or elated, or sometimes has a frightening feeling like a waking nightmare. Often a young child has problems communicating any of these symptoms to an adult, who may, especially if they have never heard of migraine auras, either be disbelieving or equally frightened because they fear there is something seriously wrong with their child.

Some children will seem pale and feel clammy with a migraine, so it is often mistaken for a virus or other infection at first, especially when accompanied by vomiting. Most children with migraine will refuse all food and just want to rest. Often falling asleep and sleeping for long periods will bring about the end of an attack.

WHAT EXACTLY IS A MIGRAINE ATTACK LIKE?

I vividly remember my first attack of migraine. It happened at school, when I was 13. I was finishing a physics exam, and suddenly realized that I couldn't read the questions because there were little flashing dots all over the page. These dots were like little 'holes' which had no colour, but were just where I couldn't see anything.

Puzzled, I looked up at the examiner. I couldn't see her face; there was just a grey hole where it should have been. If I looked straight at her, I could see her hair, her body and the blackboard behind, but no face. As I looked around the room, everything I stared at directly disappeared.

I was very frightened but I didn't say anything. When the exam finished I went out of the room and down the corridor. Now the flashing dots had become much bigger, circles of flashing zigzags which pulsated in my head. I couldn't see where I was going and had to sit down. I thought that something terrible was happening to me and that I was going blind. One of my friends went to tell a teacher.

After about 15 or 20 minutes the zigzags suddenly disappeared. I felt quite dizzy and elated; I felt strange, as if I were much taller than usual or walking on air. I told the teacher about the spots in front of my eyes and she thought it was eye strain from having done the exam, which I accepted.

About 20 minutes later I began to get the headache. Within a short time it was so intense that I didn't know what to do. I went to the medical room and was violently sick. I tried to take painkillers but threw them up again. I felt as if I had food poisoning, as if my whole body was poisoned. I spent most of the day in the medical room being sick and sitting in the dark. Lying down did not help much because the pain of resting my head on the pillow was too great.

I didn't tell my mother about all the symptoms because I was afraid she would think it was something dreadful like a brain tumour. When I had a second attack she made me go to the doctor. When he told me it was migraine I was very relieved.

WHAT CAUSES MIGRAINE AND HEADACHES?

There are a lot of myths about migraine and headaches. They are not, as is sometimes thought, more often suffered by children who appear tense, neurotic or obsessive. They occur in children of all races and all cultures. Nor is there any evidence that migraine and headache sufferers are more or less intelligent than other children. However, migraines and headaches are clearly associated with stress. They do also seem to be brought on in some cases by being too long in bright sunlight, by heavy and oppressive weather, by stuffy rooms, by travelling, by staying in bed too long, and by watching too much television. They are also often caused by food allergies or intolerances, and foods with certain chemicals in them.

Today's child is often under more day-to-day stress than in the past. Typically, the modern child will have a long journey to school, often taken by stressed and anxious parents in a car, stuck in traffic and worrying about being late. After school, many children go to play schemes or are taken from one activity to another: music lessons, after-school clubs, sports. Many children have to take competitive exams at a young age to get into the school their parents have chosen for them, with some children having to take several exams for different schools to guarantee them a place.

The pressure of modern life is relentless. Children feel they have to see the latest film, get the latest computer game, have the most action-packed birthday party yet. Many children spend hours in front of television or computer screens watching fast and furious images with bright colours and flashing lights. Far less time is spent today in a leisurely walk home from school or pottering in the garden or at home for hours. Today's child is not allowed to be 'bored'.

Further, today's children are often not allowed to be ill either. With both parents often working outside the home, children who are ill are dosed with paracetamol and antibiotics so that they can carry on and the parents will not have to take time off work. Long periods of convalescence after measles or chicken pox are a thing of the past; measles, like many other childhood diseases, is prevented with vaccinations, and children with chicken pox are despatched to school as soon as the spots have scabbed over. As with adults, a migraine can be the body's way of saying, 'Stop, I've had enough'. Migraine and headaches may be beneficial by actually forcing the sufferer to lie down and rest.

Emotional strain can also be a factor in migraine and headache. Stress suffered by the parents can be passed on to children. With increasing rates of marriage break-up and divorce, many children are having to deal with very stressful situations and complex emotions at an age where they cannot understand what is happening to them. Children may be suffering from bullying at school or may lack confidence and be anxious about their school performance. Boys especially may be told by parents to 'be a big boy and not cry', forcing them to repress their real emotions. Often these repressed emotions can come out in the form of violent headaches.

While formerly children were made to go to bed early, to read or amuse themselves quietly, nowadays children are allowed to stay up later, watching television or taking part in more social activities. Meals too are often more fragmented, with children eating frequent snacks between meals and eating less healthy foods. Migraine attacks and headaches are frequently linked to a longer than normal gap between meals, as low blood sugar seems to be implicated as a cause. Sugary snacks, sugary drinks and refined carbohydrates all lead to sudden surges of sugar in the blood, which then leads to a rapid 'down' afterwards.

Allergies and intolerances to certain foods, including colourings and flavourings, may also be a factor in some children. Certain foods, especially those containing chocolate, caffeine or hard cheese, seem the most common triggers for migraine.

Many parents with children who have migraine or headaches want a quick fix, something that will make their child instantly better and enable them to carry on with their normal frantic lifestyle. Unfortunately it does not work like that. Some drugs prescribed for adult migraines are unsuitable for children because of side-effects, and because, in any case, they tend to be less effective. All drugs have side-effects, and long-term drug therapy to enable a child to continue a too-fast and too-stressful lifestyle is not a good idea. A complete change of pace and lifestyle may be what is required.

Recent research has revealed new information about the causes of migraine and headaches, and there are more drug treatments available than ever before. However, it has also been found that changes in diet and lifestyle and the use of relaxation techniques can yield enormous benefits in preventing them. The good thing about headaches and migraine is that they are not ultimately harmful and that your child will bound back from each attack with renewed energy. They can of course cause damage to the child's development if he misses a lot of school or leads a semi-invalid kind of existence, as used to sometimes happen in the past, and it is this that this book will help you to avoid. In fact, a migraine or a headache can be a positive thing, in that it can help you to recognize when your child is over-tired and over-stretched and to make changes in his diet and lifestyle which will make him happier and healthier in the long run.

Today, there are many well-recognized forms of alternative or complementary medicine which can be very powerful in dealing with stress, headaches, and migraines. Rather than just treating the symptoms, these treatments deal with the causes of the headaches and can lead to long-term resolution of the problems.

This book will look in more detail at what causes migraine and headaches, how to cope with an attack, and the various conventional and complementary medical treatments available which can make your child's headaches and migraine a thing of the past.

Note: 'He' and 'she' have been used to describe your child in alternate chapters to avoid the more cumbersome 'he or she'.

Chapter One

What Causes Headaches and Migraine?

Pain in any part of the body is a sign that there is something wrong. Rather than ignoring pain, or simply taking pills that will mask the symptoms, it is important to find out the cause of headaches and try to prevent them.

A headache in a child can have many causes. These are often stress, tension, eating the 'wrong' food or illness. A severe headache or migraine in a child can be very frightening, especially the first time it happens, and many parents may fear it is something more serious. It can be important to eliminate other possibilities.

Headaches can be a symptom of illness. Many children get headaches with colds or flu or other viral infections, and with the childhood infections such as chicken pox and roseola infantum. Headaches, together with fever, are often the first symptom of flu. Severe headaches, however, can also very occasionally be a sign of serious infection such as meningitis. If your child has a headache, fever, aversion to light, a stiff neck and a skin rash, call your doctor immediately. Headache, sensitivity to sound and light, a stiff neck and nausea or sickness may all be symptoms of migraine, but a raised temperature and skin rash are not.

It is natural for parents, to whom their child is usually the most important thing in the world, to fear that there may be something seriously wrong when they are ill, especially when the pain is as severe as it is in a migraine. Some parents whose children have frequent headaches worry about the possibility of a brain tumour. Brain tumours are mercifully very rare, although they are increasing. Visual disturbances can be a symptom of a brain tumour, so it is not surprising that some parents mistake their child's migraine for something worse. Also, many children and adults get migraines on waking, which also can be a symptom of a brain tumour.

In practice, headaches are not the most common symptom of a tumour and other symptoms will be apparent to the doctor. A quick examination, looking into the back of the child's eyes, will show if there is the increased pressure inside the skull which would be caused by a tumour. It is very rare for any child who suffers from headaches or migraine to be referred for further tests.

A doctor should also be consulted if the child has a headache after a head injury, if there is a very sudden and severe headache out of the blue, or if the headache is accompanied by a sore throat or earache.

The main cause of headaches in children and adults is stress and tension, and the causes of this need to be addressed. This is particularly important with children, as the child can form habits which will stay with them all their lives. The following can all be involved in causing headaches and migraine:

- bad posture
- poor diet
- stress and tension
- lack of exercise
- allergies and/or intolerances.

Migraine is not the only form of recurrent headache. More common are the normal tension headaches caused by muscular contraction. In fact, tension headaches can occur in a sensitive person as well as migraine, in between migraine attacks or perhaps precipitating them. Because of this, it can often be difficult to distinguish between recurrent tension headaches and true migraines.

People often imagine that because children are young, supple and active and are not burdened with the responsibilities of adult life they should not get tension headaches, but this is far from the truth. As life gets more stressful, it seems that headaches in children and teenagers are becoming more common.

THE MECHANISM OF TENSION HEADACHES

When faced with stress, most people contract their muscles as if to get ready to fight, or as if they are bracing themselves to meet an enemy. Commonly the jaw tenses, the eyes screw up, the shoulders are raised and the face tips forwards. All these movements cause the muscles to go into a state of permanent contraction. When the muscles are working overtime like this, the blood cannot get enough oxygen to the contracting muscle fibres for normal aerobic tissue respiration, and so the muscles start to produce lactic acid as a by-product of what is called anaerobic respiration. This lactic acid causes the muscles to ache and feel uncomfortable.

The tensing of the muscles of the neck has other effects too. It can put pressure on the main arteries taking oxygen to the brain. This can make the sufferer feel dizzy, tired and light-headed, and often results in a headache. This tension can also prevent the lymphatic system from draining the waste products of respiration away from the tissues. Children with tension headaches often look pale due to a decreased blood supply to the face, and sometimes puffy, because the fluid cannot drain away.

Carrying heavy school bags is one common cause of headaches, especially when the bag is carried on one shoulder. This causes the shoulders to be permanently raised, putting strain on the shoulder muscles and on those of the neck. It is important to get your child a well-fitting rucksack as this distributes the weight more evenly over their back. Getting organized with homework can help your child, cutting down the numbers of books that they need to take into school every day to a minimum. You can also try to persuade the school to install lockers, although not all schools have the space.

Sitting for too long in front of television or computer screens can also lead to tension headaches. Children will often loll in uncomfortable positions on the sofa or in a chair while watching television, the programme they are watching acting as a distraction to the discomfort or pain they are suffering. Children playing with games consoles or computers often tense their muscles for long periods, hunching their shoulders and leaning their head forward. It is a good idea to make sure that children who play computer games for relatively long periods have regular breaks to do something physical in between. Breaks of 10 to 15 minutes every hour are essential; this is what is recommended in offices for adults, and is mentioned along with epilepsy warnings in the information that comes with most computer games.

In a few susceptible children, migraine headaches can be precipitated by the rapidly flashing lights or complex forms found in some computer games. Recently in Japan there was an outbreak of children having epileptic fits when a certain cartoon was shown on television; the same thing may rarely be the case with migraine.

Sinus headaches

Other common causes of headaches are sinus problems. The sinuses are spaces in the bones of the skull which open into the nose via a small hole. The lining of the nose extends into the sinuses, so infections of the nose and throat can lead to infections of the sinuses as well. A viral infection will probably just cause the cheeks to ache and produce a general feeling of heaviness and stuffiness in the head. A bacterial infection will lead to a raised temperature, bright red cheeks and often a very bad headache.

Dental problems

Occasionally dental problems can be the cause of headaches. Bad alignment of the teeth and jaw have been proved to be involved in causing headaches and migraine. Since the early 1980s there have been claims that altering the 'bite' of the teeth was successful in treating migraine. In some cases a child may have an undershot jaw where the lower teeth stick out in front of the upper, or a jaw where the two sets of teeth meet exactly, putting stress on the jaw when eating. Where fillings have not been done correctly the mouth may not be able to close properly and chewing may result in jaw movements which put stress on the muscles. This will usually need correcting.

In one piece of research, Glasgow Dental School noticed a marked improvement in patients provided with a small plastic splint to cover the upper or lower teeth when the patient was in bed. The 'splint' separated the teeth, allowing the jaw to find the most comfortable position and prevent tooth grinding or clenching which was causing headaches. The study showed the greatest benefit in those who had tension headaches rather than migraines.

An infected tooth can also cause pain which results in headaches. If your child is getting frequent headaches it is a good idea to visit the dentist to check for any problems.

Eye strain

Although most children should have their eyes tested regularly at school, sometimes short sightedness, long sightedness or astigmatism go unnoticed. This will cause the child to tense the eye muscles to try to force the eyes into focus and this can lead to tension headaches and migraines. If this is the case, wearing properly prescribed glasses or contact lenses can often cure the headaches. Again, if your child suffers from headaches, an eye test may be important to confirm that there is a problem or reassure you that this is not a cause.

WHAT IS MIGRAINE AND WHAT CAUSES IT?

Migraine and recurrent headaches are so common that a great deal of research has been undertaken to find out what causes them and, if possible, to develop a 'miracle cure'. Despite all this effort, however, the actual nature of migraine is still unclear.

What is clear is that migraine is not 'just a headache'. Physiological changes take place in the whole body, but no-one knows why. Migraines arise in the hypothalamus in the brain. This is an extremely complex structure at the base of the brain which controls functions crucial to survival such as temperature regulation, heart rate, blood pressure, feeding behaviour, water intake and emotional behaviour. The hypothalamus also includes the reticular activating system, which consists of reticular cells which extend from the central part of the brain stem to all parts of the cerebral cortex, determining the amount of stimulation which is allowed to reach the brain.

ANATOMY OF A MIGRAINE

The prodrome

Migraines are usually preceded by what doctors call a 'prodrome', which can occur one or two days before the migraine proper. This involves first of all a change of mood, causing elation or depression. Children may typically become highly excited and irritable and charge around, or they may become extremely short-tempered and frustrated. Some children will become floppy and lethargic, and complain of extreme tiredness or an aching-all-over feeling similar to the beginnings of flu. They may yawn a lot and become floppy, or they may become clumsy and accident prone.

Many children and adult sufferers of migraine also experience a carbohydrate craving in the day or two before an attack. This may be the body's way of trying to raise the blood sugar level. Sometimes a child may crave chocolates or other sweet things and these may then be blamed for the migraine attack when it starts, although this craving is a symptom of the attack rather than the cause.

The aura

Perhaps the most striking and bizarre aspect of a migraine is the aura. Migraine aura occurs in about 30 per cent of migraines, but is more common in children than adults. The existence of the migraine aura was one of the main factors which led doctors to think that migraines started in the brain and were a malfunction of the nervous system. The fact that epileptic fits are also preceded by a prodrome and aura led people to make a connection between the two conditions, a fact which still causes people to worry today (see page 12).

Migraine auras can be bizarre and frightening, especially the first time a person experiences them. The main symptoms are disturbances in vision which are usually very typical, but there can also be other sensory disturbances such as disturbances in smells and sounds, a change in mood, disturbances in speech, dislocations of time and space perception, and dreamy and trance-like states. Your child may seem confused, may stumble, be unable to talk or jumble up her words, or may go blank and stare into space. Very occasionally there may be numbness or paralysis of the limbs.

Visual disturbances

The most common 'hallucinations' are visual ones. The simplest of these are brilliant stars, sparks or flashes (called phosphenes) which may dance, drift or flash across the visual field. Another common symptom is 'holes' in the vision. These often start small, and may appear in the centre of the visual field, so that the child cannot see what she is looking directly at. It is a bit like the effect of being dazzled by the sun or by a photo flash bulb. Often these holes become bigger, advancing across the visual field, and at the margin there are often brilliant lights, either white or with bright rainbow colours. Some people see geometrical shapes similar to those found in Turkish rugs, with squares, zigzags, and honeycombs.

The whole effect usually scintillates rapidly, at a frequency which has been estimated at 8 to 12 scintillations per second. The expansion of this phenomenon – known as a migraine scotoma – seems to take about the same time in all migraine sufferers, too, about 20 minutes from the first appearance to disappearing off the edge of the visual field.

More rarely, children and adults get other hallucinations too. Some people may smell something that isn't there. Other people become very sensitive to smells which they wouldn't normally notice. Some hear sounds. Some find that their limbs tingle or go numb, and others can't control them properly. Some people have a sense of almost unbearable elation, similar to a religious ecstasy. Indeed, some writers believe that the visions of some medieval saints were migraine auras. Others have a sense like a waking nightmare, or a sense of 'nameless dread'.

Sufferers from migraine also often say that at this stage in the migraine they feel as if they are being bombarded with sensory information. Food tastes more strongly than usual, sounds are louder, colours are brighter. The body is in a state of arousal. This is followed by a state of depression as the migraine progresses. Some writers have even described migraine as 'a disorder of arousal'.

All these symptoms can be very frightening and confusing to a child, who may also find it difficult to explain them to an adult. People who do not know about migraine auras may think that their child is making things up. Some children and adults actually enjoy the aura. The visual hallucinations can be very beautiful and the emotional high so rewarding that some migraine sufferers would actually prefer not to suppress them, despite the headache which usually follows.

The headache

After the aura comes the migraine itself. The headache is, of course, the main symptom. The usual description is that the pain is heavy, throbbing and involves the whole head. Sometimes it is referred to as 'stabbing'. Some people cannot bear to move their head; others cannot bear to lie down because of the pain caused by the pressure of the head on the pillow. Movement usually aggravates the headache, as do bright lights and sounds. Typically the sufferer wants to retreat to a quiet, darkened room.

The word 'migraine' comes from the Greek words *hemi* and *crania*, meaning half the head. Migraine headaches are often described as being one-sided, and this is sometimes the case; however, some people think that their headaches cannot be migraine because they are not one-sided. In fact it is more usual for the pain to involve the whole head. It may also involve the face, jaw, neck and shoulders.

The headache is caused by the contraction of the blood vessels inside the skull. In a migraine preceded by the aura, there is a reduction in the blood supply flowing to the brain. The brain requires a certain amount of blood to function normally, and when the blood supply falls too low, symptoms occur. The first symptoms usually occur in the occipital lobes at the base of the skull, which control vision, causing the visual disturbances typical of a migraine aura. If the blood supply drops further forward in the brain, numbness and weakness of the face, arms and legs may occur.

Following this, the blood vessels to the brain expand. When

an artery becomes distended, this stretches the surrounding nerve fibres which send out messages of pain. With each pulse of the heart, the fibres will fire, giving the characteristic throb of migraine. On top of this pain is the pain caused by the tensing of muscles in response to the arterial throbbing.

It used to be thought that this contraction and dilation of the blood vessels was solely responsible for the pain of migraine. However, it is now known that the problems with the blood vessels are likely to be caused by the neurotransmitter serotonin. Serotonin – its chemical name is 5-hydroxytryptamine – seems to act to inhibit the passing of nerve impulses. Its actions have been implicated in sleep processes, in pain and in depression. Messages are passed along nerve cells through electrical impulses. However, in between the nerves, the messages have to be transmitted on to the next nerve cell across the cell walls through a chemical process. This depends on the neurotransmitters, chemicals released at the nerve junctions and which either speed up or slow down the transmission of impulses. Serotonin is one of these neurotransmitters.

For a long time researchers have been working with the idea that migraine sufferers are somehow wired up in such a way as to be more sensitive to outside stimuli, which can trigger changes in the brain. During a migraine attack they appear more sensitive to pain, and the migraine attack may be caused by the abnormal firing of nerves in the brain which signal pain.

Serotonin appears to be involved in this process. However, it also acts in many places in the body – a fact which may explain the whole body being affected during a migraine. Serotonin appears to be released into the bloodstream before a migraine attack. Blood platelets – tiny cells which circulate in the blood and which clump together to form clots when blood vessels are damaged and help in the repair process – are known to release serotonin and one theory is that people who suffer from migraine have 'leaky' platelets.

Other theories under investigation involve the build-up of

chemicals in the brain which have to be discharged, resulting in a migraine – this would account for the cyclical nature of migraine attacks and the fact that there is a period after a migraine in which you cannot have another one.

Most migraine sufferers also experience feelings of nausea, sickness or feel 'liverish'. Some children – and adults – may also experience loose bowel movements or diarrhoea. This aspect of migraine was known about in ancient times and was partially responsible for migraines being put down to 'an excess of yellow or black bile'. The modern interpretation is that serotonin is also involved in smooth muscle contraction and thus the action of the gut. What exactly the links are, however, remains unknown.

The resolution

Eventually the migraine headache will resolve. Some migraines last for hours, others for as many as two or three days. With children, most migraines are of shorter duration, and they often resolve with vomiting, crying, or the child falling asleep.

The hangover

After a migraine, many people experience a 'hangover' in which they feel tired, listless and extremely sleepy. If your child is allowed to sleep this off, he will often wake up bouncy and refreshed. Adults often say their system feels 'cleaned out' or purged. A burst of energy may follow the migraine.

The refactory period

There is what is known as a refractory period after a migraine, in which it isn't possible to have another migraine. So, many people are also relieved that in the days after a migraine they can't be about to get another one.

Not all children or adults go through all these stages. The majority of migraine sufferers do not experience an aura. The prodrome or hangover afterwards may be less intense in many people. In children, particularly, the attacks seem to be shorter, and this, together with the fact that some children find it difficult to explain what they are feeling, means that child-hood migraine may be difficult to recognize.

Case Study

When Amelia was six she had these strange episodes. She would be her usual self in the morning, full of energy, playing and running around and asking millions of questions. Suddenly she would go quiet, look a little pale, and yawn a lot. She would say she felt funny and had a tummy ache, and would refuse to eat and sometimes say that she felt sick. Usually she would go and lie down; unusually, she wouldn't want to watch TV or listen to a tape because she would say it was 'noisy'. She would go to sleep for a long nap – about two hours – and then wake up refreshed.

Amelia's migraines were not properly diagnosed until she was 11 years old.

Migraine and epilepsy

Many doctors and writers in the past have linked migraine and epilepsy, although the stigma against epilepsy and the severity of the condition in some cases have led others to suppress the possible connections. The fear of epilepsy has also been responsible for some of the fear attached to migraines. Doctors have pointed out that there are similarities, for instance epileptic fits are often preceded by a prodrome or aura. However, the migraine aura is usually very characteristic and different from that which occurs before epileptic fits. Visual symptoms are far commoner in migraine, and the classic scintillating patterns described above are never found in epilepsy. However, the mood changes in the prodrome, with its profound experiences of elation and terror, are very similar.

Very, very occasionally a migraine attack is accompanied by a brief loss of consciousness. Doctors are undecided as to whether this is a variation of true migraine or whether in these instances an epileptic episode has been superimposed on a migraine.

Epileptic fits do seem to be very slightly more common in migraine sufferers, and vice versa. Migraine does also appear to be slightly more common among people who suffer from depression in later life and migraine is a very small increased risk factor for strokes. However, this is a small increased risk – from 2 to 3.6 per 100,000 at age 20 – and strokes are extremely rare in children.

Interestingly, doctors investigating migraine have looked at brainwave patterns through doing an EEG (electro-encephalogram) examination, in which electrodes are placed on the head to measure the brainwaves. Despite the large numbers of these studies, no clear pattern has been found. Some researchers claim to have found 'spikes' in brainwave activity at certain frequencies in between attacks, but no clear pattern has ever emerged that would enable a doctor to diagnose migraine on the basis of an EEG. This is quite different from the situation in epilepsy, where distinct abnormal EEGs form the basis for diagnosis.

EEGs are, however, frequently abnormal during a migraine attack. Some doctors and researchers have described a migraine with aura as being similar to a very slow epileptic fit. Unlike epileptic attacks, however, there is no possibility of resultant brain damage.

▓ INHERITING MIGRAINE

There is no doubt that there is a genetic component in migraine. If parents or other close family members have suffered from migraine, a child is more likely to. However, twin studies do not show a huge genetic factor. It is probable that the *tendency* to have migraines is inherited, but that there are many factors involved, rather than the inheritance of a single gene.

One of the most reliable and careful studies of migraine and inheritance was carried out in 1954. Researchers studied 119 people who suffered from regular migraines and found that 28.6 per cent of those in whom neither parents had migraine were sufferers, 44.2 per cent of those with one migrainous parent had migraines, and 69.2 per cent of those with two migrainous parents had migraine. The genetic link seems to be stronger with classical migraine (migraine with aura), and there is one form of migraine known as familial hemiplegic migraine where the inheritance pattern is very clear.

However, these studies do not take into account the fact that families provide role models for children and that factors other than genetic ones which make migraine run in families might be involved. Recently, interest has been shown in the idea that children may *learn* how to have migraines from the example of others. Since the child is laying down nervous pathways in the brain, this pattern of response may become fixed. Trying to do something to prevent this pattern from establishing itself while your child is young is therefore important for preventing migraines later on.

Research carried out in the United States in 1996 shows that many migraine sufferers have inherited bad habits in managing their migraines from older family members. Nearly half of the participants in one survey said that their strategies for dealing with headaches were influenced by adult family members. More than three-quarters said their mothers had the greatest influence. The survey showed that 59 per cent of sufferers went to bed,

57 per cent took over-the-counter medicines, 8 per cent tried to ignore the symptoms, and 3 per cent took 'home remedies'. While more migraine sufferers today take prescription medicines – 44 per cent as opposed to 19 per cent – the most common strategies reported by younger migraine sufferers were also going to bed and taking over-the-counter medicines.

Many children with migraine have parents who suffer from migraine too. If the mother's attitude is to 'grin and bear it', then the child may feel they have to do the same. Parents with migraine may just feel it is something that can't be helped. A parent who 'worked through their migraines', feeling unable to take time off, may expect their child to do the same. They may delay taking the child to a doctor or doing anything to change the symptoms because they are unaware that new understanding has made it easier to deal with and prevent migraines.

Just as some children copy their parent's response to migraines, others react against it.

Case Study
Joanne had suffered from migraines since she was 13. She had them every month before her period and would go to bed and lie down in a darkened room for two days. Nobody in the family was allowed to make any noise and her daughter Kelly had to get supper for her younger brothers.

When Kelly became a teenager she, too, used to suffer from migraines. Her mother said that it was just something she had to put up with. However, Kelly went to the doctor and was prescribed painkillers which helped her and enabled her to carry on with her usual activities.

The 'migraine personality'
It used to be thought that certain personality types were more likely to suffer from migraines. The typical child with migraine was seen to be rigid, over-achieving and 'sensitive'. This view is now thought to be false. Different children, whether introvert or extrovert, placid or temperamental, all suffer from migraine. There is some truth in the fact that children who are under

stress may be more prone to migraine; parents who want their child to achieve highly at school or who over-stimulate their child may be responsible for driving them too hard, stressing them out and causing them to suffer headaches and migraines.

Another theory is that migraines are the result of emotional repression, that the migraine is a way of the body releasing suppressed anger, conflict, fear and hostility. The fact that many adults and children who are migraine sufferers find relief after psychotherapy has shown that there is some truth in this. If there have been problems in the family, such as the death of a close relative, a divorce, a house move or other stressful events, it may be worth investigating some kind of counselling for your child or your whole family.

If your child suffers from migraine it is important not to stigmatize your child as 'delicate'. If you say they are delicate and over-sensitive this can become a self-fulfilling prophecy.

THE MECHANISM OF PAIN

Pain is a very complex phenomenon and its nature is still not entirely understood. It is known that people's emotional state can have a great bearing on the amount of pain they suffer. Anticipating pain can be worse than pain itself, as can be seen when adults or children dread having an injection or visiting the dentist. Victims of torture often say that the fear of being hurt and not being able to control what happens is worse than the actual physical pain itself.

Throughout the body there are pain receptors which, when activated, send nervous messages to the brain. (Interestingly, there are no pain receptors inside the brain, although there are in the membranes and blood vessels which surround it.) However, the brain has to receive and interpret these signals. Many painkillers, such as the opium derivatives, morphine, codeine, and so on, actually do not stop the pain but stop the brain from minding about the pain. The brain can ignore nervous impulses selectively if it wants to. If you are at a noisy party and want to concentrate on a fascinating conversation you're having with someone, your brain will shut out most of the noise around you. The brain can also shut out regular or familiar sounds, like the ticking of a clock or the humming of a fridge.

The brain stem is responsible for deciding which signals go through to your conscious mind and which don't. There is now a theory that there is a kind of 'gate' in the brain which only allows pain signals to go through when it is open. It is known that in the heat of battle even severe injuries are sometimes not noticed until later, presumably because this 'gate' is closed at the time.

It is thought that in some people this mechanism may not work well. Some research has shown that migraine and recurrent headache sufferers find sounds uncomfortable and then painful sooner than those who never have headaches. Migraine sufferers find that during an attack all external stimuli – temperature, light, sound, taste, touch – are too strong. Their pain gates may be open when it is not necessary.

LOW MAGNESIUM LEVELS

Magnesium is an essential mineral which is needed for many metabolic processes. A diet high in refined and processed foods is often short of magnesium.

Some researchers have been investigating whether low magnesium levels could be responsible for causing migraine. Some studies have indicated that migraine sufferers have low levels of magnesium in their bloodstream and saliva, and that the blood serum levels tended to be reduced further during attacks. Some doctors have suggested that magnesium supplements might help, but this has not been proven.

Food sources rich in magnesium include:

- nuts
- shrimps
- soya beans
- whole grains
- green, leafy vegetables.

Tap water in hard water areas also contains magnesium. You can get magnesium supplements, but these act as a laxative and too much can lead to diarrhoea.

THE WEATHER

It may surprise some people that headaches and migraine can be caused by the weather. Research has shown that migraine sufferers are often very sensitive to changes in the weather. In Canada, one study showed that migraines were more common during close, wet, stormy weather. High pressure and clear, sunny weather seemed to cause fewer headaches and migraines.

Cold weather and icy winds may cause people to hunch their shoulders and tense their jaws, thus causing headaches. Hot, dry winds also seem to cause headaches, perhaps because of positive electrical charges in the air. Migraines are common before a thunderstorm.

The presence of negative ions from trees and running water can be beneficial to migraines.

Migraine triggers
Most people who suffer from migraine discover that certain events act as 'triggers' for their migraines. The most common migraine triggers are:

- delaying a meal/skipping breakfast/lunch
- eating certain foods (eg cheese, red wine, caffeine-containing foods, chocolates, fizzy drinks)
- spending time in a stuffy, smoky, noisy atmosphere
- sleeping in late
- stressful events such as exams

- menstrual periods
- bright light or flashing lights such as disco strobes
- certain smells (commonly gloss paint, varnish, tar, dry cleaning fluids and petrol)
- bright psychedelic zigzag patterns
- violent exercise
- emotional states such as anger, anxiety, aggravation and annoyance

Avoiding these triggers can mean that the child with migraine can lead a comparatively migraine-free existence. In fact, the clue to coping with most migraines and headaches is through changing your child's or your family's lifestyle.

In addition, many alternative or complementary therapies can deal with the actual causes of migraine and headaches and can often prevent or even cure the problem.

Chapter Two

Diet and Lifestyle

It has long been known that there is a link between diet and headaches and migraine. Most people are familiar with the effects of over-eating and of drinking too much alcohol, and in fact many of the symptoms are exactly the same for migraine; headache, lack of energy, nausea and feeling 'liverish'. It seems that there may be substances to which the migrainous child or adult is particularly sensitive, and these are found in many of the foods that children (especially teenagers) and adults over-indulge in.

For a long time people have known that certain foods seem to trigger migraine. Among them are:

- chocolate and cocoa
- hard cheese
- blue cheese
- coffee (or other drinks like cola which contain caffeine)
- preservatives, such as sodium nitrite which is added to pre-cooked meats such as bacon, ham and salami.

All the main triggers of migraine, such as stress, hunger, fatigue and certain foods, are associated with changes in the body of substances called 'vaso-active amines'. Chocolate contains one such amine, betaphenylethylamine, while tyramine, histamine and phenylethylamine are found in alcohol and some cheeses. The catecholamines, noradrenalin and adrenalin, are released under stress and when the blood sugar level is low. These amines are broken down in the body by a group of enzymes called the monoamine oxidase enzymes; research in the past has suggested that migraine sufferers may be short of these enzymes. This enzyme system is also affected by the hormonal changes in a woman's menstrual cycle and the hormones in the contraceptive pill, both of which are known to be linked to migraine in women.

Evidence is now emerging that foods and inhaled substances can actually cause both headaches and migraine. However, it is still not clear whether these changes are the cause of migraine attacks or simply part of the pattern of migraine once it has started.

As mentioned before, cravings for certain foods are often part of the early signs of a migraine attack, and so, people often crave chocolate or other foods and then blame this for the migraine. If your child loves chocolate or cheddar cheese then it can be very hard always to forbid it. If your child genuinely seems to be sensitive to one of these foods, then it can help to limit your child to small quantities, or only to give your child these foods after a migraine attack, when he is unlikely to have another one. You should certainly make sure they avoid such foods when a migraine is 'due'.

■ FOODS AND DRINKS USUALLY AVOIDED

In a study of 494 people with migraine at the Princess Margaret Migraine Clinic in London, UK the following proportions of people avoided the foods listed below because they thought they precipitated migraine.

Alcohol	29 per cent
Chocolate	19.2 per cent
Cheese and dairy products	18.2 per cent
Citrus fruits	11.1 per cent

The types of food and drink within these categories varied. Some people find they can drink some types of alcohol, such as white wine, but not red. Some can drink in the evening but not at lunchtime, and some say that certain drinks – sherry, brandy, champagne – bring on attacks while other forms of alcohol do not.

With dairy products, cheese is the most common trigger, with people saying that the more matured cheeses or blue cheeses are most likely to provoke an attack, with the most frequently mentioned being Stilton, Brie, Camembert and Emmental.

Among fruits, citrus fruits are the most commonly mentioned. Other foods that are also often mentioned include yeast extracts (Marmite, Vegemite), fried fatty foods, onions, some red meats and pickled herring. Soy and peanuts are also fairly frequently cited as migraine triggers.

Ice cream is another food which is frequently mentioned as a migraine trigger. Ice cream is of course a dairy food, and is very rich and high in fat. It is also very cold, which may be a factor. Further, ice creams are often eaten on hot, bright, sunny days, often in the fresh air when a child has been exerting himself. The combination of all these factors may make ice cream a sure trigger for a migraine attack.

Alcohol
Although most people would be horrified to think that young children were regularly drinking alcohol, a recent survey showed that a surprisingly high number of children were offered alcohol at parties and other social events. Some of these were as young as toddlers. The marketing of alcohol-containing sweet drinks aimed at teenagers has meant that many children as young as 10 or 11 are consuming alcohol regularly. Teenagers are often under heavy pressure to consume alcoholic drinks at parties or to pretend they are old enough to buy drinks in bars and pubs.

Alcohol is a known trigger for migraine and headaches. Red wine seems to be the most likely to cause problems, along with brandy, sherry and port; this is because these contain complex alcohols called congeners which are known to be involved in hangovers, as well as tannins and other substances. White wine, or clear spirits like vodka, seem to be less problematic.

Clearly it is not a good idea for children or teenagers to consume more than a very little alcohol. Children need to be told about the dangers of alcohol and that it is addictive, and that excessive binge drinking can lead to unconsciousness and death. If your child suffers from migraine, alcohol is best avoided altogether.

EATING REGULARLY

More important perhaps than the danger foods is the danger of not eating regularly or developing low blood sugar levels.

People seem to vary in their need to eat regularly. Some people can go like mad all day on half a cracker for breakfast and not seem to notice. Many people are not that extreme, but can vary mealtimes and eat large or small meals without experiencing any problems. Some people, however, seem very sensitive to fluctuations in blood sugar levels and need to eat regularly. These people become rapidly tired, irritable, weak, headachy and unable to concentrate if they do not eat regular meals.

Migrainous people seem to be in this category, and this is particularly noticeable with children. Most small children will become very tired and irritable if they miss a meal. In fact, it has been shown that the biggest trigger for migraine attacks in children is not what they ate beforehand, but not eating beforehand.

Food cravings

Another confusing factor is that in the prodrome to migraine, many children and adults have food cravings. They may suddenly want to eat chocolate or some sugary and starchy food. Then, when the migraine proper begins, they may blame that food for causing it, not realizing that the migraine had already been triggered before they had the desire to eat.

DIETING

Many children today are excessively conscious of their weight. Even primary-school-age children can be heard to talk about dieting and losing weight in the school playground and are often quite cruel to those who are seen as 'fat'. Surveys have shown that a majority of teenagers interviewed would 'like to be slimmer'. Unfortunately, many children and teenagers decide to 'diet' without any information or advice about how to go about it. Many skip meals such as lunch, and then, when they become ravenous in the mid afternoon, are tempted to have unhealthy snacks which probably contain more calories than a proper lunch. Skipping meals and going short of food is a frequent cause of migraines, and many children who try to diet are cutting down on the vital nutrients they need.

If your child is overweight and needs to diet you should help them to do it slowly. Cutting down on refined carbohydrates and sugary foods over a long period will cause weight loss and will also help prevent migraines. If your child wants to diet, you should consult your doctor or a dietician to work out a healthy and nutritious diet which will help your child lose weight without becoming hungry. Your whole family may also need to change their eating patterns.

Rapid dieting and skipping meals is likely to cause no weight loss and is likely to lead to worse headaches and migraines.

Hypoglycaemia

A constant supply of glucose is needed to provide energy for the cells which make up the body. The body keeps the glucose level stable with two substances, insulin and glucagon. Glucagon releases glucose from the liver where it is stored as glycogen, and insulin takes glucose out of the bloodstream and converts it to glycogen to be stored.

Hypoglycaemia is the result of glucose levels in the body falling below the required level. Hypoglycaemia is increasingly common, partly due to Western habits of eating far too much starchy and sugary food. When large quantities of glucose hit the bloodstream, large quantities of insulin are released to mop it up. Often too much is released in response to these excessive quantities and too much glucose removed. Adrenalin is then released in response to low blood glucose levels, causing the person to become aggressive, sweaty, pale and trembly.

The best way to deal with this problem is to eat a diet which will release sugars into the blood slowly. This means, on the whole, a healthy diet with a mixture of protein-rich foods, fresh vegetables and wholemeal breads and grains.

Foods can be measured according to their glycaemic index on a scale of 0–100. Pure glucose would score 100. The glycaemic index reveals how quickly each food raises the blood sugar level.

The glycaemic index reveals some interesting facts. Some breakfast cereals which contain sugar, white bread, potato and white rice are absorbed very quickly and raise blood sugar levels very fast. The 'healthy' foods to eat are those with a glycaemic index (GI) of 50 or less. The table below lists some common foods:

Food	GI
Baked potato	85
Basmati rice	76
White bread	70
Muesli bar	61
Brown rice	58
Baked beans	48
Porridge	42
Apple	36
Yoghurt (plain)	33
Lentils	29
Milk	27

▨ FIBRE

Fibre is important in the diet because it helps avoid constipation and enables toxic substances eliminated in the waste to be removed from the body quickly and efficiently. Many people have made a connection between headaches and constipation, and for some people it is undoubtedly true that the two are connected. Straining to pass a bowel movement can also raise blood pressure and cause headaches. However, some degree of constipation often occurs before a migraine, to be followed by loose bowel movements and sickness, so this may be a result of migraine rather than a cause.

Fibre in the diet also helps food to be digested more slowly, preventing large fluctuations in blood sugar. A high-fibre content is part of a good diet and should always be encouraged. Good foods are:

- oats (porridge, flapjacks, fruit crumble with oat topping)
- fresh vegetables and fruits
- wholemeal bread
- dishes with lentils or other pulses.

▨ A HEALTHY DIET

The increasing numbers of pesticides, fungicides, preservatives, sweeteners, flavourings, colourings and other additives in food may be a factor in the increasing number of food allergies. These artificial chemicals may combine with the natural foodstuffs to produce an allergic response, which may be a factor in causing migraine and headaches.

Even when your child is trying to follow a healthy diet, there can be problems. Many foods we eat are contaminated with chemicals. Fruits are sprayed with pesticides and fungicides. Apples and lemons are often coated with paraffin wax to improve their shelf life and appearance. Green bananas are ripened artificially with ethylene gas. Corn is soaked in sulphur dioxide to prevent fermentation. And so on. If your child is sensitive to any of these, eating organic produce may be necessary.

It goes without saying that your child will be less likely to develop allergic conditions if he eats a healthy diet, with fresh fruit, raw or lightly cooked vegetables and freshly prepared foods. Organic meat, organic milk and dairy products and organic vegetables are available in specialist shops and in an increasing number of supermarkets.

Studies have shown that today's children tend to eat far too many processed foods, with a diet high in crisps, chips, fried foods such as cheap burgers and fish fingers, and sweetened and salted baked beans or spaghetti hoops. Many children prefer white, refined bread to wholemeal alternatives, and many popular breakfast cereals have a high sugar content. Children also eat large quantities of biscuits, chocolate bars, sweets and fizzy sweet drinks. In addition, many processed, frozen and ready-made meals have been cooked for long periods which remove many of the vitamins necessary for health.

FOODS FOR OLDER CHILDREN AND TEENAGERS

Older school-age children and teenagers often become very fussy about their diet, and are often influenced by their peer group and by 'in' foods advertised on television. As a parent it can help if you cook healthier versions of popular foods such as burgers and pizzas. Many teenagers become concerned about animal welfare and the environment and their idealism can be harnessed in helping them to understand why it is important to eat healthy foods such as organic meat and milk and vegetables, and that this benefits animals too. Concern about keeping slim can also be used to help teach your teenage children the importance of a healthy diet, although today's children are often so afraid of becoming fat that they go short of food, and this can trigger migraines.

Food additives
Children with migraine should, whenever possible, be given fresh foods. Convenience foods should be as free from additives, preservatives, colourings and flavourings as possible, as these may provoke a reaction in a sensitive child.

Food additives will be listed on the label as E numbers. Not all E numbers are harmful; E160, for instance, is carotene, a naturally occurring colouring present in carrots.

The groups of additives which are believed to aggravate migraine particularly are the azo dyes and the benzoate preservatives. There are 11 azo dyes, the most common of which are tartrazine (E102), sunset yellow, (E110), amaranth (E123) – a red dye – and ponceau 4R (E124) – green. Others are E107, E122, E128, E180, E151, E154 and E155. There are ten benzoate preservatives with number E210 to E219. Some children are undoubtedly sensitive to these chemicals and they have been linked to hyperactivity, poor sleep and headaches.

Eat little and often

Migraine and headache sufferers on the whole seem to do better when they eat little and often. This helps to keep the blood sugar level constant but also means that the child is not over-loaded with one kind of food. Migraine and headache sufferers should eat small, starchy snacks and avoid sugary foods. Healthy snacks, such as muesli bars or sandwiches, are better than confectionery and crisps. A good breakfast – a high-fibre cereal with milk, or porridge, or yogurt, and wholemeal toast – is a big help.

Some school lunches are not very healthy. If your child seems to be getting a lot of migraines, it can help to change to a packed lunch where you can control what goes in. At school, a child may be eating a very high fat and high sugar diet. The staple is often mashed potato or chips, pizza made from white flour is popular, and there is also white bread, and starchy puddings to follow. Wholemeal bread sandwiches, carrot sticks or celery, muesli bars or flapjacks, a yoghurt and fresh fruit makes a much healthier lunch and will sustain your child for longer too.

You can give your child break-time snacks for school – muesli bars or a piece of fruit. It can also be important to give your child a healthy snack as soon as he comes home from school. If your child has after-school activities, it is important to give him a snack to have after school, especially if he will be taking part in some sporting activity which will burn up calories. Give your child their evening meal early – about 5.30 or 6 pm rather than waiting to have the main evening meal until your partner comes home from work at seven or later.

A bedtime snack is also a good idea for the child who tends to wake up with a migraine. This needn't be large – a piece of wholemeal bread or toast and a milky drink or a bowl of cereal is fine.

Your child should never go more than four hours without eating – preferably not more than three. A small child should eat even more frequently.

▦ FOOD ALLERGIES AND INTOLERANCES

There is a difference between allergy and food intolerance. The term 'food allergy' is normally used when the child has a dramatic or obvious reaction to eating a food which occurs soon after touching or taking it. For instance, developing a rash around the mouth or more generally soon after taking the food, or being sick, or having a more severe response such as anaphylactic shock.

The term 'food intolerance' is used when the reaction to a food is less clear-cut, and may occur some hours or even days after the food is taken, so is often 'masked'. Most masked food allergies involve staple foods which the child consumes every day, such as wheat and dairy products. With a masked food allergy, the child develops a tolerance for the food and may even crave it. If the food is withdrawn and then reintroduced four or five days later, an allergic reaction can normally be noticed.

For a long time the medical establishment was fairly sceptical about food intolerances, but it is now accepted that these can cause symptoms such as the following:

- eczema
- asthma
- headaches
- migraines
- digestive problems
- chronic fatigue
- irritability.

Allergy tests

It can help, if you suspect a food allergy, to have your child allergy tested. This can be done in a variety of ways.

Patch test

This involves deliberately placing potential allergens onto an area of skin, usually on the back or arm. Each patch is covered with a plaster for 24 to 48 hours and then the skin is examined. If there is a reaction on the skin, an allergy is suspected. However, the tests are not always completely reliable.

Skin prick test

A solution is made up containing small quantities of the potential allergen, and this is introduced into the skin by pricking with a sterile needle. If the child is allergic to the substance, there will be a slightly raised lump or weal 15 minutes later. Because most children are afraid of pricks or needles, however, the patch test is usually preferred.

Kinesiology

Kinesiology can be used as a diagnostic test for allergies. Samples of possible allergens are placed, one by one, on the body. The practitioner then exerts gentle pressure on the arm. If the subject can resist then they are not allergic, but if the muscles in the arm weaken, there is an allergic response.

Exclusion diet

Another way of testing for allergies is through an exclusion diet. This is difficult to achieve with a child, but it is the most reliable test. The classic elimination diet requires fasting for four days, at its strictest taking only pure mineral water. Since this is not really feasible with children, and starvation is likely to provoke a severe migraine, the child is normally given three foodstuffs which almost never provoke an allergic response; lamb, pears and rice. Other foods are introduced one by one to see if they cause a reaction. It may take over a week of giving larger amounts of the potential allergen before a response is seen, and this needs to be repeated for different foodstuffs. It can take weeks to find out which foods are responsible for your child's migraines and/or headache, if any.

Rotation diet

Here, suspect foodstuffs are given at a minimum of every four days; often five works better. You give your child a different meat for each day, a different fruit, a different drink, and so on. You must keep a record so that if a reaction occurs you can check what foods caused it. To make it easy to see which foods are involved, avoid complex cooked and ready-made foods which contain many ingredients.

Some doctors are sceptical of the food allergy approach. However, in a 1983 study at Great Ormond Street Hospital for Sick Children in the UK, an impressive 93 per cent of the 88 children who took part showed some improvement in their migraines after following an elimination-type diet.

Common allergens

The most common allergens in the modern diet appear to be:

- cows' milk and other dairy produce
- tomatoes
- citrus fruit
- yeast-containing foods
- wheat
- coffee
- chocolate
- food additives.

Avoiding all these would make it very difficult for you to give your child adequate nutrition, but fortunately very few children are allergic or intolerant of all of these.

It is also very important not to become too obsessive or faddish about food with a young child. Children need a wide range of nutrients to meet their needs and also a very strict diet can be monotonous. With a child who suffers from headaches or migraine, the problem is often to get the child to eat more food more frequently, so strict diets don't necessarily help. If you are going to try an exclusion or elimination diet you may need the help of a doctor, dietician or complementary therapist to work out a menu that will provide all your child's needs. *The Elimination Diet Cookbook* (see Further Reading, page 101) will show you how to do it but with a young child in particular you should never attempt it on your own.

■ KEEPING IT IN PROPORTION

It is also important to resist the temptation to be over-protective of your child if he has migraine or recurrent headaches. You should allow your child to do what other children do as much as possible. Dietary restrictions can have important consequences for a child, as in our culture food is symbolic of other things. Food is seen by children as a way that parents show love for the child. If you withhold treats or foods your child likes, he will often think you are withholding love. Similarly, if your child has food which is 'different' from other children, this can create social difficulties. If a would-be friend offers your child a Mars bar, seeking friendship, and he refuses it, the child will feel rebuffed. He will probably not understand that your child cannot eat it. Food restrictions can make social occasions, school meals, visiting friends and going to parties a bit of an ordeal for your child. He may turn down invitations to go to a friend's house for supper because he is afraid he won't be able to eat the food, or be reluctant to ask a friend back as they will see what he eats at home.

It is also not always easy to know what is going on outside the home or between children. One child's mother found that her son was swapping his home-made cakes and biscuits for shop-bought confectionery in the school playground. He would also swap sought-after football stickers for sweets. Further, it is very difficult to cut some foods out of a diet. You can cut out the obvious sources of cows' milk such as milk, yoghurt, ice cream, cheese and butter, but it is not always realized that many margarines contain skimmed cows' milk or whey, or that many biscuits, soups, and pre-packed meals contain milk products.

Depending on the severity of the reaction, it is probably best to waive the normal rules occasionally, as with children's parties.

Case Study
'We used to send Thomas to parties with a little box of his own "safe" foods,' recalls his mother. 'We were trying to avoid wheat, dairy products, citrus fruits and chocolate. It was only when I went to a party early and saw him standing on his own in a corner nibbling at a sandwich while everyone else was sitting round the table eating crisps and chocolate cake that I realized he was missing out socially. We decided it was sometimes better to let him enjoy himself and then suffer the headache than never enjoy himself at all.'

Chapter Three

Helping Your Child

In many cases it should be possible to prevent headaches or migraine or reduce the symptoms. However, often this can only be done by making significant changes to your child's and your family's lifestyle.

Keeping a migraine diary

One of the most useful things you can do is to keep a migraine diary. You should keep a record of:

- what your child eats
- what time he or she wakes up and goes to bed
- any particular stresses, excitement or exertion
- any weather changes.

With a teenage girl you should also keep a record of the menstrual cycle. You should then make a note of when your child has a migraine and see if there is a pattern and whether you can identify a particular trigger factor. Sometimes the triggers will be clear and obvious, sometimes not. Often a migraine seems to be an accumulation of a number of factors rather than one isolated cause.

SLEEP

There are several links between sleep and migraine. First, scientists know that the chemical messenger serotonin involved in migraine is also involved in sleep. There are two stages of sleep:

deep sleep and REM or Rapid Eye Movement sleep, in which dreaming occurs. Young babies fall into REM sleep first and then shorter cycles of deep sleep; older children and adults fall into deep sleep with patches of dreaming sleep. Children dream more than adults.

There is an increase in the blood supply to the brain during REM sleep. Studies have suggested that migraine sufferers experience a higher level of brain activity at this time. It is also known that sleeping can often stop or resolve a migraine attack.

A well-known trigger for migraine is disruption of sleep patterns. Too little sleep, and getting overtired, will often lead to a migraine attack. Many parents will find that their child can get away with one late night, but two or three late nights in a row, such as when away from home, is usually followed by a migraine. On the other hand, many children get a migraine when after a week of getting up early in the morning to go to school they have a long lie-in on Sunday. If this happens regularly, try waking the child up half an hour after the normal school-day wake-up time, then an hour after, then a bit more, to see how much extra sleep your child can tolerate. If your child seems to be going short of sleep and needs to catch up, try getting them into bed earlier rather than allowing them to go short of sleep all week and then trying to catch up at the weekends.

Jet-lag is also likely to cause migraines, and many people who get migraine are very sensitive to jet-lag or changes in time zones. Some are even upset by the small change twice a year when the clocks go forward or back an hour. If your child suffers from regular migraines, it is important to make sure not only that they get enough sleep, but also that they have a regular routine where they go to bed and wake up at much the same time every day. This can cause a tremendous reduction in the frequency of headaches.

It can also be important to make sure that your child goes to bed in a calm and relaxed state. It can help if your child gets her homework out of the way earlier in the evening so that she can relax later in the evening, and packs her bag for school early in the evening so that she is not running around late in the evening trying to prepare for the next day, and doesn't go to bed worrying about homework that hasn't been completed or where she has left her sports clothes. Having a relaxing bath before going to bed can help and it is certainly a good idea to try not to have rows or start conversations about important issues at bedtime.

REDUCING POLLUTION IN YOUR ENVIRONMENT

Pollution and the chemicals in the environment which surround us nowadays may be a factor in the increase in headaches and migraines. If your child suffers from headaches or migraines it is important to try to reduce the number of chemicals in your home environment as much as possible.

- Avoid using perfumes, deodorant sprays, cleaning agents and perfumed soaps.
- In the garden, cut down on fungicides, pesticides and other chemicals.
- If you need to decorate, do it in the summer when all the doors and windows can be open and when decorating your child's room, move the child into another room to sleep until the paint is completely dry.

There have also been concerns about the increase in electrical equipment in the home and the possibility of magnetic fields having an effect on the body. It is impossible for most people to put the clock back and live in an environment without these things, especially as radio waves permeate everything. You can, however reduce the level of electro-magnetic exposure by turning off electric blankets, televisions and computers and ensuring that clock radios and televisions are not left near your child's bed. If you live on a busy street, fumes from traffic can also be a problem. Not everyone has control over where they live, but if your child suffers from migraines or recurrent head-aches, it may be an idea to avoid living near high tension power lines, near a busy main road or on the flight path to a major airport.

TRAVEL SICKNESS

Children who suffer from migraine are more likely to be carsick, or suffer from 'motion sickness'. Such children may be seasick or sick on airplanes too. Antihistamines may be prescribed for travel sickness, and can help with migraines (see page 54). Some researchers have pointed out that many migraine sufferers had travel sickness as a child, and children who suffer in this way may be more likely to suffer migraines later on.

If your child suffers from travel sickness, try breaking up the journey, having lots of short breaks, giving your child things to eat and drink, and keeping her eyes focused outside the car – perhaps by playing 'I Spy' or seeing who spots the most red or blue cars. Such strategies will also help prevent headaches and migraine on long journeys.

HOLIDAYS

One sad fact is that holidays can often be hell for the migraine sufferer and their family. Travelling can be a real problem, especially if meals are missed or there are stresses such as running late. Jet-lag can induce migraines, as can lying in the sun on a hot beach. Too much sleep, too little sleep, a glass of wine (red wine is often a trigger for migraines) and changes in routine also predispose young people to migraine. Also, the fact that migraines often happen after a period of stress means that as soon as the child starts to relax and enjoy themselves, the migraine hits them. A change in diet can also add to the problem.

Holidays can also be a stressful time for other reasons. Often it's the only time in the year when the family spend so much time together, and issues that are swept aside much of the time can surface. Family stresses and tensions often come out, resulting in rows and emotional upsets. You can help your child by putting thought and careful preparation into your holiday.

- Don't neglect your child's diet while on holiday.
- Try to keep to their usual routine as much as possible.
- Make sure they do not stay in the sun too long.
- Don't let them stay on the beach so long they miss lunch or supper.
- Try to avoid situations in which they could yet stressed; organizing in advance can help reduce tension.
- Take emergency supplies in case flights are delayed.

EMOTIONAL PROBLEMS

It has been shown that children who suffer from emotional problems are more likely to get migraines and other recurrent headaches.

These stresses are not the only factor, however. The frequency of migraines and headaches also seems to depend on the way the child deals with stress. Many people think that blocking or repressing emotions felt in response to the stresses is most likely to provoke migraines. When we are tense or worried we tend to contract our muscles, frowning, tensing the neck, raising the shoulders. If the emotions are not released, this tension builds and builds until a headache or a migraine results. This is not to say that migraines are 'all in the head', but it is clear that the stress and tension caused by unresolved emotional difficulties can lead to headache or migraine. This is often the case when there are family difficulties such as marital discord, when a child is under too much pressure to achieve at school or at home, when they are worried about bullying or not fitting in at school, or when they have other pressing difficulties.

Boys are particularly vulnerable to hiding or blocking their feelings, because of the mistaken idea that 'big boys don't cry'. In fact, crying and the release of tension involved often seems to help with migraine attacks. Hitting a pillow and getting rid of anger can also help. Encouraging your child to admit to their worries and express their feelings can also be of benefit.

Case Study

'Ben was nine when he started getting migraines. There was a lot of stress because my husband and I had been getting on very badly and there were lots of rows. In the summer my husband moved out, then he came back to have another go at the marriage but that didn't work out and we separated officially in the spring and started divorce proceedings.

'Ben was very quiet but he was very attached to his father and I know he blamed me for the divorce. On the surface I was doing most of the shouting and he didn't see the whole picture, and I didn't want to seem to run his father down by putting my point of view. He started doing badly at school and kept complaining of tummy aches and headaches.

'Eventually the headaches got so bad we went to see the doctor who said that it was migraine. The doctor recommended that he saw a counsellor. Ben didn't want to go at first but we said it would only be for a few sessions and in fact he liked the woman he saw and he did seem to cheer up a bit. I think it helped that he still saw a lot of his father and actually things settled down a lot. He still says he wishes we could get back together but he's much more settled and the migraines have got much better.'

Sometimes, particularly with teenagers, parents have to admit that they are the last person their child wants to confide in. If this is the case, it can help to find another adult, perhaps an aunt or a friend, or perhaps some kind of therapist or counsellor, with whom your child can share their worries. It is fascinating and true that almost every family has its secrets and areas which they do not talk about. It is also true that family members need some privacy from one another, and this is particularly true in the teenage years when the child is trying to make an emotional separation from the parents and discover their own personality, needs, and feelings. An over-anxious or over-involved parent can cause as many problems for a child as the parent who isn't there or doesn't care.

A research paper published in the journal *Headache* in February 1996 looked at a random sample of 113 schoolchildren aged 8 to 15 who had a headache once a month or more. This showed that children who suffered headaches had more stress and complained of tiredness and 'difficulty in relaxing'. They were also more likely to complain of 'eye tiredness', 'feeling chilly', to have poor appetites and breathing problems. Schoolchildren with headaches seemed more stressed by having many leisure activities.

Headache sufferers were more likely to have other kinds of pain, such as stomach, back and neck pain. They felt more tired, though they were not having less sleep. They were more likely to be absent from school and experience less satisfaction with school. In clinical samples, children with migraine had more self-reported somatic complaints, anxiety, and depressive symptoms, than the control group of children who did not have headaches or migraine.

This study doesn't show whether these factors were a result or a cause of migraine. However, it is clear that children with migraine can suffer a great deal in various ways in addition to the suffering directly caused by the migraine or headache itself.

Many children today are also under great pressure from the

stress of school examinations, and very competitive entrance examinations.

Case Study

Amy was ten when she started getting severe migraines. She had suffered from 'sick headaches' before, but only two or three times a year. Amy was very musical and was learning violin and piano. She had music lessons two evenings a week and went to the Centre for Young Musicians on Saturdays. She also went to a French club and swimming class after school and on one night she had lessons with her tutor as well. Amy's mother was very keen that she should do her Grade 5 violin exam as this would help her to get a music scholarship and help with entry to a very selective school.

Amy's mother realized that everything was becoming too much and that her daughter was more in danger of messing up her school entry through having a migraine than by not practising enough. She dropped French club and decided to leave the swimming classes till after Amy's exams. She also arranged for the violin lesson to be at a slightly later time so that Amy could eat her supper beforehand. Amy seemed to become much less stressed as soon as she had some time at home on her own, messing about and doing nothing in particular. She started sleeping better and the migraines became less severe and less frequent.

PHYSICAL EXERCISE

Regular though not excessive physical exercise can be very beneficial for children who have migraine and/or headaches.

Exercise is physically tiring and also relaxing. In addition, it seems to help the release of endorphins, the body's natural painkillers, which are responsible for the feeling of well-being many people experience after physical exercise. Exercise also helps promote a healthy tiredness and restful sleep.

Excessive exercise, or exercise which causes a child to miss meals or results in low blood sugar levels, should be avoided. Make sure your child knows how to pace herself and to take breaks rather than pushing herself to the extreme. Some sports, such as cross-country running, should probably be avoided. Always make sure your child has snacks before, sometimes during, and after exercise.

Case Study

'Sebastian started getting migraines when he was seven. Eventually when he was 12 the headaches had started to interfere with his schoolwork; he frequently had to go and lie down in the medical room and several times I was called away from work to go and pick him up -- he was so ill he couldn't possibly have made his own way home. We got a referral to the City of London migraine clinic and they told us to make sure that he went to bed on time and got enough sleep, that he ate a bowl of nourishing cereal at bedtime (sometimes he used to wake up with migraines) and that he avoided sport. One of the problems was that he was in the school football team. They had practice at lunchtime which hardly left any time for him to have lunch and certainly not a sit-down lunch in the canteen – and then he would have a match after school. Most of the suggestions were helpful, but of course he could not be persuaded to give up football, so we just try to drum it into him that he has to eat before and after a game.'

VDUS, TELEVISION, AND ARTIFICIAL LIGHTING

Glare and flicker from computer and television screens and fluorescent lighting can cause headaches and migraine in sensitive children. Make sure that you have a low-glare screen for your home computer. Sitting some distance from the television screen can help. If your children watch television or play on a games console or computer, make sure that they take frequent breaks – at least ten minutes in every hour, as recommended, but ideally much more. Eye strain if your child is too close or too far away from the screen can also cause tension headaches.

It is known that intense flashing light at certain frequencies can trigger epileptic fits in sensitive children. It is possible that these can cause migraine headaches in some children too. Flickering fluorescent tubes can also trigger migraines. Check the lighting in your home and replace old or faulty bulbs or tubes.

FAMILY SUPPORT

Support and sympathy from family, friends and staff at school can be essential for the child who has migraine. The presence of a parent soothing and holding the child can help enormously. Your child may need reassurance that nothing very serious is wrong and that nothing terrible is going to happen to her.

Unfortunately, many people do not react with sympathy, even within the family, especially when people are busy and routines have to be changed and activities curtailed. Parents may be called away from work, trips postponed and outings cancelled. If a child has migraines often, the usual first reaction of everyone is 'Oh no, not another migraine!' This is very hard on the child, as the last thing she wants herself is another headache.

It is important to realize that your child cannot help getting migraines. Sometimes parents may blame their child for going to bed too late, eating the wrong food or for 'working themselves up' into a migraine. It is very hard for an adult to exert such self-control – imagine how much harder it is for a child. Blaming your child can only make her more miserable and will add to the stresses which result in migraine.

A much more helpful approach is simply to sympathize, provide warmth and security, and try to remove causes of stress until your child has recovered.

HELPING OTHER CHILDREN IN THE FAMILY

When a child has an illness or a disability, it can sometimes seem to other children in the family that this child is taking precedence over the others. Siblings may feel that the other child is 'special', having special foods cooked for them, having extra visits to the doctor or migraine clinic, and receiving extra attention. They may not realize that their parents are trying to compensate for the things the child is missing out on.

Children are always looking out for signs that the parent is giving more love and attention to one child than another. When the whole family is together, try to treat them all equally and try not to draw attention to the child's special diet. Try to make sure that the whole family eats more healthily and follows the same kinds of routines.

MIGRAINE PRECAUTIONS

You can help your child by taking precautions to prevent or deal with a migraine attack.

- Always take food with you in case you are delayed.
- Take painkillers in case they are needed.
- Have a first-aid box in the car.
- Relax. Try to avoid your child getting wound up if you are late.

To abort an attack:

- encourage your child to sleep if at all possible
- give them a snack or sugary drink
- try giving them a hot or cold shower or a bath
- relax and soothe your child.

■ NATURAL PAIN RELIEF

If your child is in pain, there is a lot that you can do to ease their pain without resorting to drugs or painkillers. With migraine, painkillers are not always effective anyway, and your child will benefit from any other support you can give.

When a child has a migraine, the support and understanding of the parents and other people around them can help enormously. The presence of a caring parent soothing the child and holding her hand can help the child relax and speed recovery. Soothing and stroking a child really does help to ease pain. Relaxation helps relieve the tense muscles which result from the headache and which can make it worse and also prolong it. Hands are known to be healing, and the 'laying on of hands' is a time-honoured way of relieving pain and helping sickness. Healing of this sort works because the person believes the healer can help. Who is more powerful to a child than its parent? We all know that when a child has cut or hurt herself 'kissing it better' often satisfies her completely. Rubbing or stroking your child's head, or giving a drink to 'make it better' will often help. All these things also show you acknowledge their pain, that you care and empathize with them.

Distraction can also help. Talking to your child, reading to her in a soothing voice, and giving her something to look at can help. Your child may try to distract herself with rhythmical rocking movements or by saying the same thing over and over again; do not try to restrain her if this seems to help.

Children frequently interpret illness and pain as punishment for wrong-doing. It can be important to reassure your child that this is not the case and that it is not her fault that she has a migraine.

HELP AND SUPPORT FOR PARENTS

Looking after young children is exhausting and demanding for any parent, and looking after a child who is frequently ill is even more demanding. If a child has migraine or recurrent headaches, the parents may get trapped in domestic routines which they believe will help prevent them, and feel that no-one else will be able to do this so well. They may resist the child staying with friends overnight or visiting relatives because of special diets or routines. They may also fear that the stress and excitement of being away from the family home or of separation from the parents will trigger a migraine or headache.

While routines are important in preventing migraine and headaches, it is important that the parents get time away from the children and to relax and enjoy themselves. Going out together regularly, perhaps one night a week, can help a lot. If you are a single parent, it can be even more important to have a break. Stress and family disharmony will certainly not help, and sometimes it is necessary to take a step back to get a clearer perspective on life.

Relaxation techniques
Adults as well as children can benefit from relaxation techniques. If your child's migraines or headaches are caused by stress, there's a good chance that you, the parents, are stressed out too. Yoga and relaxation classes are often available locally at very little cost. There are also other therapies available such as flotation, in which you are immersed in a warm bath of salty water, the lights dimmed, and you drift away, listening to music or not as you choose, in a deeply relaxing, back-to-the-womb experience. Aromatherapy massage, visualization, hypnosis and meditation can also help to relieve stress and enable you to cope much better. Find out which works best for you and treat yourself whenever you can – if you are less stressed it will help your child and, indeed, the whole family.

Chapter Four

Conventional Treatments

If your child suffers from regular headaches or migraines it is a good idea to see your doctor, who can eliminate the possibility of your child having anything more serious and reassure you, as well as suggesting treatments. In recent years, a great many new medications have come on the market which may be more or less successful in the treatment of migraines. However, many of these are not suitable for use by children under the age of 12.

Before going into the specific drug treatments on offer, it is important that you discuss their benefits and side-effects with your doctor. The thought of a young child taking powerful medications for any length of time is something that you would only want to consider after all other avenues have been tried and after talking over carefully all the risks and benefits. Your doctor will often be the most helpful person, as he will know your child's background and family history. However, if your child's migraines are severe and the doctor is not able to or has exhausted all the medical treatments at his disposal, it may be helpful to get your child referred to a migraine clinic. These are specialized clinics which may either be self-contained or linked to the neurology departments of hospitals.

Your doctor should be able to refer your child. If he will not for some reason, be persistent. Your doctor may think there is nothing they can do that he can't, but the doctors in a migraine clinic have a specific interest in migraine and will know about all the most up-to-date research and treatments.

Many migraine clinics will see someone without a referral when they are experiencing an acute attack. Your child will then have the benefit of getting the best possible treatment together with a great deal of sympathy. In fact, if your doctor is not being helpful it may be worth taking your child to the surgery when he is in the middle of an attack. Many doctors will not have had first hand experience of a migraine and may see you only when your child is well in between attacks. When witnessing an acute attack he may be horrified by the extent to which the child is suffering.

MANAGEMENT OF AN ACUTE ATTACK

Treatment for migraine consists of painkilling drugs and anti-emetic (sickness) drugs to prevent the vomiting associated with migraine and to enable the painkillers to be kept in the stomach long enough to take effect.

The most common painkiller given to children is paracet-amol, which can be given as a tablet or, more usually with children, as a sweet-tasting liquid. A sugar-free version is available. The most common anti-emetic drugs are metoclopromide or domperidone.

Parents whose children have an aura preceding the migraine can usually give them the anti-emetic in time for it to become effective. It is much more difficult if the sickness starts first or at the same time as the headache as this can prevent or slow down the absorption of painkillers.

What to do

- Take your child to a warm, dark place and encourage him to sleep. Especially with small children, sleeping will often cut the attack short and your child will wake refreshed.
- If your child cannot sleep, try putting them in a warm, relaxing bath.
- Cuddling and soothing your child may help. Some children with migraine want to be alone, others would prefer somewhere comfortable to rest in the same room as you.
- Keeping him warm with the help of blankets, hot water bottles and so on may help. On the other hand, if your child is hot and sticky, a cool, gentle sponge-down can help.
- Remove stress as much as possible. Don't allow your child to feel guilty for missing an important event. Many children hate to feel they are missing out on things so reassure them that it doesn't matter and you'll make up for the missed activity another time.
- If your child asks for a drink, a few sips of a sweetened drink will help. If he is being sick don't give food – don't even mention it!
- Give painkillers as recommended every four to six hours until the attack subsides, or give homeopathic or other medicines as recommended.

SEVERE ATTACKS

Very occasionally a severe migraine attack will result in a child being admitted to hospital. This is usually because the parent or doctor is taken aback by the severity of the child's distress and may suspect some other cause. However, sometimes in a prolonged attack the vomiting can cause the child to become dehydrated and the child may need an intravenous drip to replace body fluids.

In the US, intravenous prochloperazine – a major tranquillizer – has been given for acute migraine headaches in a paediatric emergency department. The physicians reported a 90 per cent response with 'minimal adverse effects'. However, this should only be considered as a last resort.

▓ DRUGS FOR MIGRAINE

Originally, drugs were obtained from plants and animals and consumed in their natural form. Nowadays most are made synthetically but have the same or similar structure to naturally occurring forms. Many drugs used to treat migraine come from plants. Aspirin (acetylsalicylic acid) comes from willow bark, codeine from the opium poppy, *Papaver somniferum*, and ergotamine from the fungus ergot.

No drugs are completely safe, and you need to weigh up the risks against the benefits in each case. It is a good idea to start your child off with the simplest drugs first and progress to more powerful drugs only if the migraines are intolerable or disrupting too much of your child's life. There are many changes you can make to your child's diet and lifestyle which can help, as can complementary therapies, and powerful drugs should only be used as a last resort or to break a pattern of particularly frequent or vicious migraines.

Drug names
Many people are confused by the number of different drugs available. Every drug has its generic name – this is not the chemical name of the drug (which may be enormously long and unpronounceable) but the official medical term for the active ingredient. These names are usually given by doctors and written on the prescription. However, drugs are made by different drug companies and also have a brand name. With some much-used non-prescription drugs, such as aspirin and paracetamol, there may be many different names in use by different companies for the same drug, which will be packaged

differently, may be a different colour or shape and may be in a different form (soluble, insoluble, as a tablet, syrup, capsule, powder, and so on).

So aspirin is the generic name, acetylsalicylic acid is its chemical name, and it is sold under a wide number of trade names by the many different companies which manufacture it and package it in different forms.

Migraine drugs often contain a combination of different pain-killing ingredients and may also contain anti-histamines or other anti-nausea drugs.

Some drugs are available over the counter, while others can be prescribed only by a doctor.

Tips about taking drugs

- Always read the instructions and never give your child more than the stated dose. This is especially important with small children. If the instructions say take one or two tablets, start with one and see if that works before giving a higher dose.
- If you are going to give your child painkillers, do so as soon as the headache starts. Some people make the mistake of leaving it until the headache is really bad, when the medicine is likely to be less effective.
- Pills taken before food will be more effective than those taken after.
- Ask your doctor if the drug is prescribed in suppository form for a small child who is vomiting. Drugs taken by this route also work more quickly than those that are absorbed by the stomach.

Over-the-counter painkillers

Aspirin (acetylsalicylic acid)

Aspirin is one of the oldest painkilling drugs, and also lowers temperature and lowers blood pressure. However, it can irritate the lining of the stomach and lead to stomach ulcers. It is not recommended for use by children under the age of 12 because of the very slight risk of a rare condition called Reye's syndrome which affects the brain and liver and can be fatal. It is important not to exceed the stated dose. It is also unwise to give your child aspirin if he tends to suffer from allergic reactions or suffers from asthma.

Paracetamol (acetaminophen)

Paracetamol is the painkiller most commonly used by children and is available as a syrup as well as tablets. Paracetamol also lowers the body's temperature. If the correct dose is taken it is very safe. However, an overdose of paracetamol can be exceedingly dangerous as it can lead to irreversible liver failure. It is very important to keep the medicine out of the reach of children and not to allow your child to dose themselves.

The dose for children aged 0 to 6 years should be 120–240mg every six hours. From the age of 6 to 12, the dose should be 250–500mg every six hours. Look at the bottle, measure carefully and do not exceed the stated dose.

Ibuprofen

Ibuprofen is a newer painkiller which, like aspirin, should be avoided by those with allergic conditions. It can also irritate the stomach lining and cause nausea.

Codeine

Codeine is a painkilling drug related to morphine and is also derived from the poppy. It is available over the counter in low doses, often combined with aspirin, paracetamol or both. Codeine is also available on prescription in higher doses. It can cause drowsiness, nausea and constipation and can, in larger doses, lead to dependence.

Caffeine

Caffeine is used in some migraine preparations as it causes the blood vessels to dilate and can give a 'lift'. However, you shouldn't give your child a migraine preparation with caffeine in it if you want him to rest or if he suffers from hyperactivity.

Anti-sickness drugs

Metoclopramide is often used for migraine as it reduces nausea and vomiting and enables painkilling drugs to be absorbed. It may cause constipation and in large doses may cause drowsiness. It is available only on prescription.

Metoclopramide is available as a suppository, a syrup, or paediatric liquid. The normal dose is:

Age 1–3 years	1mg 2–3 times daily
Age 3–5 years	2mg 2–3 times daily
Age 5–9 years	2.5mg 2–3 times daily
Age 9–14 years	5mg 3 times daily

Domperidone has similar effects to metoclopramide but is less likely to cause sedation.

Buclizine and **cyclizine** are anti-histamines which can cause drowsiness and reduce nausea.

Some migraine remedies contain a mixture of different drugs. By checking the contents you will be able to know what drugs they contain, such as an anti-emetic, pain reliever, and sometimes caffeine.

More powerful prescription drugs for migraine

Ergotamine

Ergotamine tartrate is one drug used to treat migraine, but, it is not often used for children because it takes at least 30 minutes to get into the system, often doesn't work, and can have unpleasant side-effects.

Over the years ergotamine has been much prescribed for severe migraine. It constricts the swollen blood vessels and reduces pain. However, it should be used with caution because of its side-effects. It is very important not to take more than 6–8mg of ergotamine for any one migraine attack, and with children a much smaller dose, about a quarter of the usual 2mg per dose, will suffice. It can be chewed or swallowed or given as a suppository. You cannot repeat a treatment within a week. The side-effects can be unpleasant, including nausea and vomiting, trembling, pain and muscle cramps and cold hands and feet. Ergotamine can also cause rebound headaches, which are mistaken for migraine, causing the sufferer to take more ergotamine, and so on.

Serotonin-related drugs

Pizotifen is a preventive drug used for those who suffer from frequent and long-lasting migraines. It is an anti-histamine as well as anti-migraine drug and can cause nausea and drowsiness as well as more serious side-effects such as increase in appetite and weight gain, dizziness, flushing of the face, muscle pains and mood changes. Pizotifen should be taken every day and should start to take effect after two weeks.

Each tablet contains 0.5 or 1.5mg of pizotifen, and the syrup contains 0.25mg in each 5ml. The dose for children should be from 0.5–1.5mg at night.

Methysergide is sometimes used for the treatment of severe migraine in adults but has so many serious side-effects that it should only be given under strict medical supervision.

Sumatriptin is the latest drug developed specifically for the treatment of migraine. It is thought to affect the serotonin receptors in the brain which control the constriction of blood vessels. If taken at the onset of an attack, it can completely abort it, and if there is the warning aura it can prevent the headache from occurring at all. However, in some people the drug simply delays the migraine by 24 to 48 hours.

Sumatriptin has not been in use long enough to be certain that it is safe for children so it is not prescribed for children under 12.

Beta-blockers

Beta-blockers are drugs used to treat high blood pressure and anxiety. However, they have also been found to prevent migraines in some people if taken regularly. A three- to six-month course may be all that is required to break the cycle and make the migraines less frequent.

Beta-blockers can have unpleasant side-effects, including cold hands and feet, dizziness, nausea and depression. They should not be used in people suffering from asthma or diabetes. Because of their effect in slowing the heart and reducing blood pressure they cannot be used on people with heart or circulatory problems. They are not normally recommended for use by children, although older children can be treated with them.

Propranolol is the most commonly prescribed beta-blocker. The normal dose for adults can be quite high, from 40mg three times a day to treat anxiety disorders up to 360mg a day in divided doses to treat high blood pressure. However, according to Dr Anne MacGregor of the City of London migraine clinic, as little as 10mg twice a day should prevent or reduce the severity of migraines.

All the drugs listed above can have unpleasant side-effects and can cause health problems when taken frequently over the long term. In addition, some of the drugs cause dependence and some of them may actually lead to headaches when treatment is stopped. For children who may suffer from migraines for much of their childhood and adult life it is clearly important to avoid the use of drugs whenever possible, and to concentrate on dietary and lifestyle changes which can be equally effective in reducing the frequency and severity of migraines.

Fortunately, it is becoming increasingly recognized that many of the 'alternative' or 'complementary' treatments are of great benefit in treating migraine. If you are already seeing a complementary health practitioner, this can be your first port of call. If not, and you have tried the various drug treatments available without success, you might consider looking into the alternatives listed in the next chapter.

■ INVESTIGATING HEADACHES AND MIGRAINE

The first thing your doctor will want to know is when your child started having the headaches or migraines, how long they last, how often they recur, and exactly what the symptoms are. With an older child, the doctor will usually talk to the child directly. With a young child, however, the doctor will need to ask you about the symptoms and may need you to interpret what the child does say. Many children are quite awed by the experience of seeing a doctor. They may not be able to express themselves clearly. Young children in particular find it hard to describe or locate pain adequately.

If migraine has been diagnosed, there are various drug remedies. Most doctors will start with the mildest first, then use stronger medicines or preventative measures if these do not help.

For children, in an acute attack, paracetamol or ibuprofen

are recommended – not aspirin for children under 12. This can be given as a syrup or tablet or, if a child is being very sick, as a suppository. In some countries suppositories are given very frequently, in others people are often reluctant to give them, which is a great pity, as they can be of great benefit in migraine as they act more quickly and also won't be vomited up again. You can buy disposable plastic gloves if you aren't comfortable with doing this. An anti-emetic drug can also be given by suppository on a 'milligramme per kilogramme of body weight' basis.

One problem with drugs and young children is that the child can't choose, and some parents tend to over-prescribe as a matter of course, while others try to avoid giving all drugs, which, if the drugs don't cause bad side-effects, can cause their child to suffer unnecessarily.

Case Study
Clio's parents first became worried about their daughter when she was two-and-a-half. 'This coincided with the birth of her baby brother. She started having stomach upsets which became more and more frequent and usually resulted in her being repeatedly sick. The "sicky bouts" usually started in the late afternoon or early evening and were usually all over by 11 o'clock. They were more likely to occur at the weekend and happened about every month to six weeks.

'After two or three of these episodes I took her to the doctor, but because she was always better by then, he didn't think it was a problem and seemed to think this was quite common and she would grow out of it. I talked to the health visitor who thought that these bouts might be some form of attention-seeking behaviour caused by jealousy over her brother, so for a while I tried to ignore the attacks and give poor Clio as little attention as possible.

'Soon, however, it became clear that she really was ill and in pain, and she started to complain about headaches. We gave her paracetamol syrup but she hated the taste and always sicked it up within about ten minutes of our giving it to her.

The headaches became more frequent and we were beginning to worry that there might be something seriously wrong with her.

'Eventually we called out the doctor while she was having a particularly bad attack and at last he recognized that it was migraine. Once he told us that, everything fell into place although no-one in our family had suffered from migraine before.

'The migraines have not gone away, but now we know what they are we have some control over them. If Clio complains soon enough, I always give her something to eat and often that stops it. If not, I give her paracetamol and put her straight to bed (the migraines usually happen in the early evening anyway). If I put her to bed soon enough she usually just sleeps them off and wakes in the morning fully recovered. I try to limit her activities so that she doesn't get over-excited or over-tired.

'Sometimes Clio tries to take advantage by saying she's got a headache when she wants to get out of something she doesn't want to do such as sports at school or visiting relatives. This doesn't usually work but it makes it harder for us to know when she is genuinely getting an attack.'

Chapter Five

Complementary Therapies

A distrust of relying on powerful drugs which have side-effects and may harm the body and a desire to be treated as a whole person and not just a body with specific symptoms are two reasons why people are increasingly turning to complementary therapies.

It is clear that in the case of children with recurrant headaches and migraine, conventional medicine has little to offer other than over-the-counter painkillers. More drug treatments are on offer for teenage children, but many parents want to avoid the possible long-term side-effects. The so-called 'alternative' or 'complementary' therapies have much to offer for headaches and migraine. Increasingly, doctors are realizing that the complementary therapies can offer help where they cannot and will often support or even suggest complementary treatments.

It is difficult to prove the benefits of many complementary therapies because the role of the mind is so important in dealing with illness. Most complementary therapies are 'holistic', that is, they involve the mind and the emotions and the patient's personality and temperament as well as their body. It has been shown that 'placebos' – tablets or injections which the patient believes to contain a drug but which don't – can be highly effective in relieving even severe pain, because the patient believes it will work and relaxes. Medical progress has been based on the idea of the 'double blind' trial in which neither the doctor nor the patient knows whether she is getting the active drug or a placebo. This is because if the patient thinks she is receiving a drug she is more likely to respond, and if the doctor believes she is prescribing a cure the patient somehow senses this and responds better too.

Human contact and sympathy and 'taking care of yourself' are also very powerful in relieving symptoms and pain. This is particularly true with young children. Most parents will instinctively 'kiss it better' when the child has a cut or bruise, and a kiss, cuddle or a soothing rub will often genuinely make the pain better. The simple process of giving something to swallow or soothing a child's forehead can make a big difference to her ability to tolerate pain and discomfort.

The therapies described in this chapter have all been used by people with migraine with success. However, it is essential that anyone seeking complementary treatments for their child for regular headaches or migraine should approach a qualified and experienced practitioner.

When you take your child to see a practitioner of a complementary therapy, in particular acupuncture or homeopathy, the practitioner will spend a great deal of time talking to you and your child, listening, and looking at your child as a complete person, rather than only concentrating on their symptoms. A trained homeopath, for example, usually spends an hour and a half on the first consultation.

Case Study
'The doctor spent ten minutes reassuring me that Ben didn't have a brain tumour and then said that all he could offer was paracetamol. When I went to see the homeopath we spent an hour and a half taking about Ben's diet, his general health, our relationship, our lifestyle. She was wonderfully sympathetic and for the first time someone seemed to understand what I was going through. She made a lot of suggestions which really helped, especially about his diet – he was a very faddy eater – and his sleep problems. I came out feeling that some-

thing could be done and he wouldn't just have to suffer for ever.'

Before choosing a complementary therapy, it is a good idea to read up about it and see whether you think it would suit your child. There are complementary medicine centres which offer a variety of different therapies, and a chat with the receptionist or one of the practitioners may help guide you towards the one which would most suit your child's age, personality and type of headache.

ACUPUNCTURE

The term 'acupuncture' means 'needle piercing' and this therapy is part of an ancient system of Chinese medicine. Acupuncture is based on the principle that health depends on the balance and flow of energy throughout the body. Moxibustion, the burning of herbs to stimulate the body's energy, is often used with acupuncture.

Acupuncture is based on the idea that qi (pronounced 'chee'), the vital energy of the body, flows through certain channels, or meridians, creating a network throughout the whole body and linking all parts together. There are 12 main qi channels, each connected to an internal organ and named after that organ. When a person is healthy the qi flows smoothly through the channels, but if for some reason the flow is blocked or becomes very weak, illness occurs. The acupuncturist aims to correct the flow of qi by inserting thin needles into particular points on the channels. The treatment lasts about 20 minutes and should not cause pain, only a tingling sensation. Because most children are afraid of needles, massage, tapping or pressure with a rounded probe is often used instead up to the age of seven.

The needles used in acupuncture are extremely fine stainless steel, and should not cause pain when inserted. Most acupuncturists treating children will use only the finest of needles, leaving them in place only for a few seconds.

The practitioner uses a number of clues to build up a diagnosis and decide on treatment. She needs a detailed understanding of the patient's lifestyle, medical history, personality, work and so on before making a diagnosis, and also looks at the way the patient walks and sits, at their facial expression, at their tongue. She listens to the sound of the patient's voice and watches their breathing, uses touch – especially of areas of their body which may be painful – and takes their pulse.

Acupuncture can be used as preventive medicine by correcting the energy before a serious illness can occur, and also to reverse illnesses by restoring the qi.

Not everyone responds to acupuncture, just as not everyone can be cured by conventional medicine. But, as many will testify, it can be highly effective.

In the Chinese system of medicine, migraine is usually seen as being connected to the liver, a very active organ which governs the free flow of energy around the body. The liver governs the muscles and is also related to the eyes. Migraines are seen to result when there is stagnation of liver qi, and often follow the path of the gall bladder meridian up the back of the neck, across the back of the skull and over the eyes.

Extensive research in China has shown that acupuncture is highly effective, and in the People's Republic of China traditional and modern medicine are equally used. In Western countries, this solid research has convinced many that acupuncture does work, and it is sometimes used for anaesthesia and pain relief in Western hospitals.

There is a code of practice laid down by the UK Department of Health which registered acupuncturists must follow. Information can be obtained from the Register of Traditional Chinese Medicine or the Council for Acupuncture (see Useful Addresses, page 103).

ACUPRESSURE

Acupressure is similar to acupuncture, but the hands, or some-times elbows or feet, are used instead of needles to stimulate the acupuncture points along the meridians. Shiatsu (see p. 83) or 'finger pressure' is the Japanese form which uses short bursts of pressure along the meridians.

ALEXANDER TECHNIQUE

The Alexander Technique uses breathing and posture to correct and let go of tensions in the body which may have gone unnoticed. Bad posture causes many common 20th-century ail-ments, such as backache, headaches, migraine and insomnia.

Even children become affected by the stress of modern life and develop excessive tension in their bodies. Children who play a musical instrument or some sports can benefit from the technique to remove the tensions which arise from the way they hold their bodies while practising and performing. The Alexander Technique uses relaxation and exercises to get rid of the tensions which can damage the body. In children who suffer from headaches and migraine, the neck muscles are usually extremely tight. Reducing the tension and adopting better posture can help the tension headaches and migraines reduce and ultimately disappear.

AROMATHERAPY

Aromatherapy has been described as the art and science of using essential plant oils as treatments. It is a holistic therapy, taking people's mind, body and spirit into account. Oils from plants have been used medicinally for thousands of years, and of course extracts of plant oils are used in modern medicines. Recently aromatherapy has gained enormous popularity.

Essential oils are absorbed very rapidly through the skin, and the oils are used in massage, in baths, and in skin preparations or compresses. The essences can be diluted in a carrier oil such as pure olive oil, or in beeswax or other cream bases, or in milk or honey. A certain amount of the essential oil is also breathed in, and the scent has an effect on the mind and thus on the body. Part of the oil is also absorbed directly and rapidly into the bloodstream via the lungs. The effect of the oils, together with a soothing massage or a gentle soak in a bath and the contact with the therapist all combine to have a very beneficial effect.

Children have a much more sensitive sense of smell than adults. They also seem to respond very quickly to the natural medicine of essential oils. However, children should use much smaller quantities of oil than adults and oils should always be well diluted to avoid any risk of the child getting drops of neat oil on the skin in the eyes or in the mouth. Children have a delicate skin which may be irritated by too strong concentrations. In addition, it is worth checking first that your child does not have any sensitivity to a particular essential oil.

Essential oils can be diluted in full fat milk, or goat's milk if the child is allergic to cow's milk and then massage on to the skin.

Bathing with essential oils can be a wonderful experience and can relieve skin problems. The appropriate essential oils (usually 1–3 drops for a child) should be added to warm water. As essential oils do not mix well with water, the bath water needs to be swished vigorously to disperse them. The child should remain in the water for ten minutes before being washed in the usual manner.

Another good way to disperse oils in the bath is with honey; one dessertspoonful of runny honey is an excellent disperser for the oil. Again, you need to swish well. Massage with essential oils is very useful for relaxing a child and for helping her to sleep. Children do not normally have any of the inhibitions about being touched which many adults have, so are very open and receptive to massage.

Another remedy is to massage a little of a mixture made of 20 drops of lavender oil and 10ml of sweet almond oil into the temples at the first sign of a migraine.

Inhalations are not safe for children under the age of 10, who may burn or scald themselves. Older children can use a vaporizer, handkerchief, or a special diffuser which can be bought from a health food shop, chemist or department store.

Recommended essential oils for use in treating migraine include:

- basil
- chamomile
- lavender
- marjoram (sweet)
- rosemary
- peppermint.

▨ BIOFEEDBACK

The technique of biofeedback has been found to be of great benefit in the treatment of recurrent headaches and migraine.

Biofeedback uses monitors to help you get feedback and measure bodily processes such as breathing rate, muscle tension and so on. By displaying this back to you it enables you gradually to learn to control these processes and learn bodily relaxation.

Common muscle tension habits which lead to headaches and migraine are frowning steadily, clenching teeth when anxious or angry, working at a surface which is too high, slouching in an armchair, watching TV when sitting or lying at a sharp angle (such as when lying in bed with the chin resting on your chest), hunching shoulders against the cold or carrying a heavy shoulder bag.

In biofeedback, monitors can be attacked to the forehead, neck, shoulders or other areas of tension, and be turned into a display or sound which will indicate the degree of tension. Then, as the person relaxes, this information is recorded by the monitors and displayed to them.

Thermal biofeedback can give information about blood flow and help the person gain control of their own blood flow. Concentrating on ways to get the blood to flow away from their brain can bring rapid relief from headaches.

Hand-warming
One particular biofeedback technique, that of hand-warming, can be very effective in relieving headaches. This technique often works well in children who find the experience of changing their body temperature through an effort of will fascinating. A small surface thermometer is taped to the hand. The child concentrates on increasing the blood flow to their hands, and watches the temperature rise on the thermometer. Increased blood supply to the hands reduces the flow to the head and thus eases headaches caused by distended blood vessels.

Biofeedback is obviously a difficult technique for very young children to learn. With older children and teenagers, however, it can be very helpful.

BIOCHEMICAL TISSUE SALTS

Biochemics is a medical system founded by a German doctor called Schuessler in the 19th century. He claimed that inner harmony could be achieved through homeostasis – a balance of the body's fluid and acid-alkali levels. This balance is easily disturbed by discrepancies in mineral and trace element levels, and small quantities of these salts can be taken to redress the balance. Biochemical tissue salts are sold in many chemists and health shops. They are safe and easy to take and do not interact with conventional drugs.

BIORESONANCE

Bioresonance is also known as Bicom resonance therapy after the machine used in this process. The Bicom machine tunes in to the electromagnetic frequencies emitted by every cell in the body. Some are in harmony, others not, and the Bicom can redress the balance. It can also be used to switch off allergic or intolerant reactions to food or inhalants. Samples of possible allergens can be placed either on the patient or in the machine and the allergy meridian monitored for fluctuations. This pinpoints the allergen and the degree of sensitivity to it. The theory is that the Bicom then inverts the disharmonic waves, amplifies the harmonic ones, and reflects them back to the body, rebalancing it. Bioresonance can be very useful in treating migraine and children often respond after only one treatment.

CHIROPRACTIC

This technique works on the principle of seeking out misalignments in the bones and then correcting them. A chiropractor diagnoses, treats and prevents mechanical disorders of the joints using his or her hands to manipulate the joints and muscles and reduce pain.

X-rays are sometimes used to help diagnose problems, though not always. The initial examination may take 20–45 minutes, with follow-up visits normally taking 10–20 minutes.

When a joint is out of place it can be restored by an extremely light yet rapid springing motion. The patient will often hear a 'click' as this happens. The effect is often dramatic and there should be no after-effects.

There are different forms of chiropractic. Daniel David Palmer founded chiropractic and his first successful treatment took place in Iowa in 1895. There is also a school founded in Britain in 1972 by John McTimoney which uses a technique called 'toggle recoil' adjustment. This treatment is ideal for children.

FLOWER REMEDIES

Flowers have been used for their healing properties for thousands of years by many different cultures, including the Australian aborigines, the ancient Egyptians, the Minoans of Crete and Native Americans. In the 1930s healing with flowers was redis-covered by Dr Edward Bach. In the mid 1970s, Richard Katz established the Flower Essence Society in California and many others have been inspired to research the healing properties of their local flora.

Flower essences are suitable for babies and small children because they are so gentle and free from harmful side-effects. It is important to get into the habit of giving your child a remedy frequently, usually two or three drops in the morning and two or three drops at bedtime, to reap its full benefits. The tra-ditional way to take flower essences is to drop them under the tongue, or you can add them to drinks such as dilute fruit juice or water. Flower essences can also be helpful when rubbed on the skin, especially the forehead in the case of headaches. You can also add flower essences to your child's bath.

The most popular flower remedies today are those developed by Dr Edward Bach, who practised at University College Hos-pital, London in the early part of this century. He believed that people's emotional and psychological problems were at the root of much of their illness, and became critical of medical treat-ments which dealt only with the symptoms rather than the whole person. Influenced by homeopathy, he developed 38 plant remedies from wild flowers.

Dr Bach recognized that worry and fear reduce the body's resistance, making a person feel under par and making them more likely to succumb to illness, and that the worry, apprehension and irritability caused by disease hinder convalescence and recovery of health.

Dr Bach made his flower essences by floating freshly picked flowers in a glass bowl of pure spring water in sunlight for three hours. He believed that the flower essence or energy transfers itself to the water which is then stabilized by mixing it with an equal volume of brandy.

Other flower essences are made without cutting the flowers; in Germany, for instance, Andreas Korte uses a cleaned half of a quartz geode filled with spring water which is placed in the field of the growing flower in the sun for a certain length of time to capture its energy.

The individual flower remedies chosen vary from person to person according to their personality and their exact symptoms. However, flower remedies used for headache and migraine include the following:

- Menzies banksia
- Clove
- Feverfew
- Green Rose
- Narcissus.

Add 2 drops each of Black-eyed Susan and Crown of Thorns for extra potency.

▧ HERBAL MEDICINE

Herbalism is the oldest form of medicine known. It is still used by a majority of the world's population, and in fact many modern, powerful drugs are derived from plants, such as the heart drug digitalis which comes from foxgloves, atropine from nightshade, aspirin which is found in willow bark, morphine from poppies and quinine from the cinchona tree.

While conventional medicine relies on extracting and purifying one active ingredient, in herbal medicine the whole plant is used, with a mixture of different ingredients which may reduce side-effects and produce a more balanced effect. Herbal remedies can be chewed, swallowed, applied to the skin, put in bath water or inhaled. Modern herbalists often prescribe herbs in concentrated liquid form, but some use elixirs, cordials, teas, pills, ointments, bath additives or poultices. You can also grow and prepare your own herbs, but since some plants can be poisonous, you should always seek advice from a qualified herbalist, especially before giving them to young children.

Herbal remedies from different countries may vary, especially since the herbs available will vary from region to region. Most herbalists warn that sometimes the symptoms will get worse at first to be followed by a marked improvement. This is normal with herbal remedies and should not cause anxiety.

A variety of herbal remedies have been used for headaches and migraine. Lemon balm or melissa (*Melissa officinalis*) has been recommended for migraines. Wood betony (*Stachys betonica*) and chamomile (*Matricaria recutica*) are good for headaches of all kinds. Lavender and pine as an inhalation is good for sinus headaches.

Marigold was once considered a specific remedy for headache. Used cold, thyme can relieve a headache, and hot thyme tea can be a relaxant and can help with tension headaches. Another old remedy is a hot footbath with mustard which draws blood away from the head to the feet. Basil, ginger, sweet marjoram, parsley, peppermint, rosemary and sage have all been recommended by different herbalists for the treatment of migraine.

Feverfew
One herbal remedy that works for even severe migraines is feverfew. Research has shown that it definitely has an effect on migraines; there is a chemical in the plant which is thought to

cut down on the release of serotonin from platelets which is involved in the mechanism of migraine. There are different varieties of feverfew, but it is only the wild sort, *Tanacetum parthenium*, which is useful in the treatment of migraine.

You can buy the plant from a herbalist or seeds of feverfew from a reputable seed merchant and grow it in your garden. It is not a fussy plant and will grow almost anywhere; it has attractive pale green leaves and small, attractive, daisy-like flowers. The leaves can be eaten raw or dried or an infusion can be made. It does have a bitter taste. Useful though feverfew is, however, its use is not recommended for children (or for pregnant women). Feverfew can also cause mouth ulcers and its use should not be continued if this is the case.

CHINESE HERBAL MEDICINE

Chinese herbal medicine is part of a sophisticated system used since ancient times. Herbs, minerals and some animal products are used to treat a wide range of diseases. The treatment is thought to restore harmony to the functions of the body, which normally means that several treatment components are given simultaneously. Unlike Western herbalists, who have a limited number of herbs at their disposal, Oriental medicine draws on a range of 4,000 herbs made up in various complex formulas. A limited number of these components are available in pill, tablet or liquid form, but most are prescribed as dried materials which are mixed to match the perceived needs of the individual patient. Because every patient is different, the herbal mix will differ from one patient to another. Usually the treatment is prepared by boiling the herbs and other dried materials with water for a specified period, straining off the liquid, which is cooled and then given to the patient.

The practitioner of Chinese herbal medicine will be looking for a 'pattern of disharmony', a way of saying someone's energy is blocked or disturbed. These patterns are recognized by a combination of symptoms, mental states, non-verbal behaviour, physiological signs and a reading of both tongue and pulses.

Vervain (ma-pien-t'ao) is a particularly effective remedy for migraine. Drunk simply as tea it can bring fast relief. A decoction of vervain, dandelion root, motherwort, wild carrot and centaury taken for several weeks should reduce the number and severity of what the Chinese call 'liverish migraines'. Rosemary (mi-tieh-hsiang) tea is also useful for tension headaches.

Drinking plenty of plain hot water during attacks is recommended, as is avoiding fatty and indigestible foods.

HOMEOPATHY

Homeopathy is the best known of the 'alternative' medicines and is growing in popularity. It is a system of medical treatment using medicine according to the principle of 'like cures like'. It was developed as a science by a German physician, Hahnemann, who noticed that quinine, which produces the same symptoms as malaria, could be used to cure it. The symptoms of a disease often show how the body is attempting to heal itself – catarrh is used to clear foreign organisms form the respiratory tract, vaginal discharges from the reproductive tract, and so on. Homeopathy is based on this observation that substances which cause certain symptoms can also be used to cure them. However, used in conventional doses many of these substances can be toxic and extremely harmful, so in homeopathy they are diluted to such an extent as to render them safe. The medicines are diluted by stages in an alcohol and water solution, and vigorously mechanically shaken in between in a process known as 'potentization'.

The potency of a homeopathic remedy refers to the extent and number of times the original extract has been diluted during the preparation. For example, Arnica 6c has been prepared by adding one drop of the original alcoholic extract to 99 drops of a solution of water and alcohol and shaken vigorously. One drop of this is added to another 99 drops of water and alcohol, and so on, for a total of six times. The higher the degree of dilution, the greater the potency.

Most over-the-counter remedies are of sixth centesimal potency (6c) which is appropriate for a beginner to use. The higher potencies (12c, 30c) should only be prescribed by a qualified homeopath.

Critics of homeopathy hold that in some preparations the original substance will have been so diluted that not even one molecule of the original substance can be contained in the solution, and therefore it is impossible that it could have any effect. Homeopaths believe that during potentization the properties of the substance being diluted are somehow imprinted into the molecules of the solution carrying it. There is no conventional scientific explanation of how this could happen, but then there are many other things which modern science cannot explain.

Some scientific studies have been carried out to try to 'prove' whether homeopathy is effective or not, but since the mind is so powerful in influencing illness this is very difficult. Many people believe from experience and observation that homeopathy does work. It certainly cannot have any harmful consequences, so is certainly worth trying even if you are sceptical.

Because homeopathy is holistic, the ill person's medical history, lifestyle, temperament and feelings will be taken into account. Because of this, there is no one remedy which will be useful for everyone; the remedy has to be matched to the person. In addition, the particular form the symptoms take will also affect what is prescribed. Because everyone is different and the homeopath is skilled at matching the individual to the remedy, you should always consult a professional homeopath if your child's symptoms are severe. Since migraine is considered a deep-seated disorder by homeopaths, it is always recommended that you see a practitioner rather than trying to treat the child yourself using remedies purchased from health shops or pharmacies.

Patients using homeopathy are often warned that their symptoms may get worse before they get better, and a 'healing crisis' is often observed. If symptoms get really severe further advice should be sought.

Common homeopathic remedies prescribed for migraine

While every child and every case is different, and two people with the same condition will not necessarily get the same treatment, there are some common remedies used for different types of headaches. Homeopathic remedies are usually given as soft tablets which dissolve quickly and easily under the tongue and are also easily crushed to give to babies, although they can also be given as hard tablets, powders, granules or capsules or in liquid suspension. It is best not to eat or drink anything but water for twenty minutes either side of taking the remedy, and to avoid strongly flavoured drinks or toothpaste which can interfere with the remedy.

Belladonna

For headaches of violent and sudden onset, often after exposure to bright sunlight or to a chill, and where there is sensitivity to light, sound and movement.

Bryonia alba (Bry.) or white bryony

For headaches which last all day and which are made worse by stuffy air. Pain is behind the eyeballs.

Gelsemium

For tension headaches or dizzy, sick headaches with band-like pressure around the forehead. Pains made worse by stress, movement, humidity, smoking, hot, sunny weather and thundery conditions.

Iris

For acute migraine attacks with blurred vision, nausea or vomiting, with shooting pains in temples, worse from coughing, exposure to cool air and mental exhaustion, and for weekend headaches.

Kali carbonicum (Kali-c.) potassium carbonate

For sharp, tearing, shooting pain above the eyes. Sufferer feels touchy and sensitive.

Kali phosphoricum (Kali-p.) potassium phosphate

For one-sided headache, worse for cold, exercise, excitement, worry.

Lachesis (Lach.) venom from bushmaster snake

For headaches which come on after sleep. Pain aggravated by sleep, heat, sunlight, alcohol, movement, closing eyes.

Natrum muraticum (Nat. mur.)

For migraine with visual disturbance, worse on waking, exposure to bright light, before or after a period, movement.

Nux vomica (Nux-v) poison nut (strychnine)

For headache which is worse on waking, with constipation and nausea. Counteracts the effect of frustration or an overheated liver caused by overindulgence in food and alcohol.

Rhododendron (Rhod.)

For headaches before a thunderstorm or where the sufferer is sensitive to a change in the weather.

Sanguinaria

For headache occurring from low blood sugar as a result of skipping meals, and for premenstrual headaches with dizziness and nausea.

▦ HYPNOTHERAPY

Hypnotherapy immediately conjures up an-image of a man in a black suit waving a watch before your eyes and then making you do things you wouldn't normally do. Nothing could be further from the truth. Hypnosis is in fact a natural state which we all experience, and is normally called dozing or daydreaming. It is not being asleep or unconscious. It is in fact self-induced and anyone who wants to can let it happen. It is experienced normally as a very relaxed, floating or pleasant feeling and you can also feel energized and alert.

Surprisingly, the ability to hypnotize yourself can be learned at a single session, although it takes practice to achieve a deep state of relaxation.

Hypnotherapy means using hypnosis to work directly with the subconscious mind, channelling its resources to achieve a positive change. The subconscious mind controls our feelings and behaviour, and often a negative cycle is set up which limits us. As soon as the first symptoms of the migraine begin, for example, the sufferer may immediately feel all the emotions of despair, depression, anger, 'why me?', 'not this again', and so on, and these negative emotions may be worse than the illness itself. Tension, stress and worry all make it harder for us to heal ourselves.

Hypnotherapy has been used very successfully to deal with pain and chronic illness. The hypnotherapist can teach a child ways of distracting herself from the pain of the headache. Hypnosis can work well with children, usually over the age of seven, as the child's powerful imagination can be harnessed. When a child has a migraine, she can imagine being in a calm and relaxed place, can imagine the pain being taken out of her head and drained into her feet.

The hypnotist can also try post-hypnotic suggestion, the technique which is most familiar from stage hypnotists. First the therapist gets the child into a deeply relaxed, trance-like state, when an idea or instruction can be planted into the child's mind. The suggestion might be: 'When your headache starts, you will put your hands on your forehead and press very gently. This will make the pain go away.'

MASSAGE

Massage of various kinds can be of enormous benefit to people suffering from headaches and migraine. Massage also releases endorphins, the body's natural painkillers. It is probably best, at least in the first instance, to go to someone who is skilled at massage, but if your child has migraine you can learn some simple massage techniques which will help relax your child and at least partially relieve the headache.

Simple massage techniques for headaches and migraine

Massage for headaches should concentrate on the head, neck and shoulders.

Working the forehead in strips

Kneel at your child's head and rest your thumbs in the centre of their forehead just above the eyebrows with your fingers around the side of their head. Slowly and firmly draw your thumbs away from the centre. Work in strips until the whole area has been covered. Your child could be sitting or lying down for this technique.

Pressing and circling temples

Press on the temples for 10 seconds with the flat of your fingers. Slowly release the pressure and then make slow, soft circles.

Base of skull pressure

Turn your child's head to one side with their cheek facing up, resting their other cheek on your hand. With your free hand, use the fingertips to push up and under the bone of the skull base. Hold, let the pressure build up, then release. Search out tense spots. Then turn your child's head to the other side and repeat.

Other massages for the face

Massage your child's scalp along the hairline. Press and circle the jaw muscles. Place your fingertips on their forehead and stroke their head down to the shoulders.

Shoulders, neck and upper back

Get your child to sit at a table. Gently squeeze and stroke the back and sides of their neck with rhythmical movements.

Massage their upper shoulders and the base of their neck with slow, firm, kneading strokes.

Exercises your child can do herself to relieve tension in the shoulders, neck and back are to stretch her neck forwards, sideways, and backwards, to circle her shoulder blades, and to do shoulder shrugs.

NATUROPATHY

The term 'naturopathy' was coined in 1895 by a New York doctor, John Shceel, but grew out of the 'nature cures' popular in Germany in the 19th century which emphasized the benefits of fresh air, sunlight and exercise. Naturopathy is widely practised in many countries and is especially popular in Germany. The theory is that a poor diet, lack of sleep and exercise and fresh air, and stress and pollution, allow waste products and toxins to build up in the body. Treatment involves dietary advice – a wholefood diet rich in organic fresh fruit and vegetables is recommended – herbal remedies, hydrotherapy massage and bodywork and changes to the lifestyle, all of which are extremely beneficial in treating headaches and migraine.

NUTRITIONAL MEDICINE

This term, or the term 'nutritional therapy', has been coined to cover the use of nutritional methods to prevent or treat disease. Much of the modern diet of highly-refined foods is lacking in essential minerals, vitamins and other nutrients. The aim of nutritional medicine is to work out what deficits there may be and add them to the diet in a way that will enable them to be absorbed and utilized by the body. It is usually best to add minerals and nutrients to the diet as they occur naturally in foodstuffs but often mineral and vitamin supplements are used. One very important nutrient for headaches and migraine, which may be recommended by a nutritional therapist, is evening primrose oil.

Evening primrose oil
Evening primrose oil has been found by some to be helpful in treating migraine. It is a natural oil derived from the seeds of specific varieties of the evening primrose plant. The oil is rich in the essential fatty acid gamma-linoleic acid (GLA). GLA is normally made by the body from the fatty acid linoleic acid which occurs widely in a normal diet.

Evening primrose oil has been recommended for the treatment of migraine linked to the menstrual cycle. Studies have been carried out into the effectiveness of evening primrose oil and have not been conclusive, with some trials showing a marked improvement in those treated with GLA and others showing no improvement. There is, however, a lot of anecdotal evidence that GLA can be beneficial for both children and adults with migraine.

Nutritional therapists may also advise you on treatments for your child's allergies or intolerances. They will normally recommend a system of eliminating any foods or inhalents which may trigger or even cause your child's headaches or migraine as well as a rotation diet to avoid any further sensitivities.

OSTEOPATHY

Osteopathy is a system of diagnosis and treatment using the musculo-skeletal system. The principle is to use gentle manipulation to restore and maintain the proper functioning of the bones and muscles. The founder of osteopathy was Andrew Taylor Still, who was born in Virginia, USA in 1928. Osteopathy is used for the treatment of problems of the spine, ligaments, muscles and bones. It improves lymphatic drainage and improves breathing and can be very effective in treating headaches and migraine.

Cranial osteopathy
Cranial osteopathy was first explored by a pupil of Still's, Sutherland. Headaches, dizziness, digestive problems/allergies and intolerances and nausea may be the effects of problems in the skull. The bones of the head or cranium are still separate in babies and young children. Disturbances in the cerebro-spinal fluid are thought to be caused by pressure on the cranial bones. Delicate manipulation of the cranial and spinal bones is used to restore the flow of fluid and ease these tensions.

Cranial osteopathy is especially effective with babies and young children. A long labour or difficult delivery may have caused distortions of the skull which may be the cause of colic in small babies. Many parents with fractious, crying babies have found that a session with a cranial osteopath leaves their baby relaxed and often fast asleep. It is also very effective in relieving headaches and migraine.

REFLEXOLOGY

Reflexology is a system of foot massage which has been practised in most ancient cultures from China to North America.

In reflexology, a gentle but firm finger pressure and a special massage technique is applied to areas of the feet and lower legs which correspond to glands, organs and parts of the body. Tensions in the body manifest themselves in the feet and hands and the consequent blocking of energy paths results in imbalance and disease. By applying gentle pressure with the hands to relevant areas of the foot, toxins can be removed from the body and circulation improved, restoring the free flow of energy and nutrients to the body cells.

Reflexology is not a diagnostic therapy but can indicate if certain organs or glands are under pressure. It can often detect injuries which occurred years ago, and also can detect weaknesses which have not yet developed into disease.

Treatment sessions usually take between 50 and 80 minutes, and the number of treatments required varies with the individual and the nature of the disorder. During treatment the patient may feel a slight discomfort on certain parts of the foot, and she may feel tired and lethargic at first, but this is generally followed by a renewed sense of well-being. Reflexology can create a deep sense of relaxation, which can encourage the body's own healing processes.

REIKI

This is an ancient Japanese therapy which is a way of connecting with universal energy to improve health and enhance the quality of life. Reiki works on the cause of the problem, not just on the outer symptoms, and treats the whole body, emotions, mind and spirit. The patient simply relaxes and enjoys the warmth of the practitioner's hands on their body. Reiki can help a large number of ailments, and because it can induce deep relaxation is particularly effective with headaches and migraine.

SHIATSU

Shiatsu is a Japanese therapy, based on the same principles as acupuncture, in which pressure is applied to the energy lines, known as meridians. Although thumb and finger pressure is mainly used, the practitioner can also use thumbs, fingers, elbows and even knees and feet.

The massage stimulates the circulation, and also the body's vital energy flow (qi, or in Japanese, ki). Shiatsu strengthens the nervous system and helps release toxins and deep-seated tension. On a more subtle level, Shiatsu enables patients to relax deeply and get in touch with their body's own healing abilities. The patient normally lies on a futon, and it is advisable not to eat or drink much before a treatment. A feeling of calmness and well-being usually follows a treatment, and many people feel invigorated yet relaxed.

VISUALIZATION

This is a technique which can help people with recurring illness or those who suffer from continual pain. It is a way of focusing the mind in such as way as to help the sufferer relax and think positive thoughts which can help ease pain or make it seem less hard to bear.

Relaxation technique
The technique of relaxation may be familiar to many mothers who have attended ante-natal classes, which often include relaxation exercises. The technique is to tense and then relax all the parts of the body in turn. Try the following exercise yourself, then teach it to your child.

- Start by lying on your back on the floor, bed or any comfortable place. Start with your feet. Wriggle your toes and feet, then let them flop. Lift your lower legs slightly and let them go. Wiggle your knee caps, then relax your thighs.
- Then go to your hands, wrists and lower arms. Clench your hands, then relax. Let your wrists go floppy. Lift up your lower arms and let them flop back. Then tense and relax your upper arms.
- Move to your shoulders. Hunch them, let them go, wiggle them until they're relaxed. Then relax your neck. Press your head back against the floor or bed, then relax again. Make sure your neck is stretched out straight and not twisted to one side.
- Then think about your face. Lift your eyebrows, let them go. Squeeze your eyes tight shut, then relax. Frown, then relax. Twitch your nose. Clench and unclench your jaw. Grin, then relax your mouth. Let your lips part slightly if they want to and your jaw sag.
- Concentrate on breathing. Take in a deep breath, let it go, relaxing your chest. Relax your stomach muscles and go on breathing slowly and steadily.

It can help to use visualization techniques to relax. Help your child relax by telling them to imagine they are somewhere lovely and soothing, such as a tropical beach with the sound of the sea in the background, the breeze stirring in the leaves above, the soft feel of the sand and the warmth of the air. Or if your child seems hot and feverish, they could think of a snowy landscape, a snowman and a Christmas tree, and floating up into the air.

With practice, this technique should rapidly induce a state or relaxation and induce sleep. It is possible to teach these techniques to children and especially to teenagers, to help them sleep off their migraine, and more generally, to go to sleep at night and to cope with stress.

PSYCHOTHERAPY AND COUNSELLING

It is not always possible to give a hard and fast definition to the difference between a counsellor and psychotherapist. There are also psychoanalysts, and many different schools of psycho-analysis – the Freudian and Jungian are best known, but there are also Kleinian, Adlerian, Rogerian and so on. There are also psychiatrists – medical doctors who then specialize in psychiatry – and psychologists, not medically trained, but people with a degree in psychology and who may specialize in educational, clinical or academic psychology. There are also behaviourists. All counsellors, psychotherapists and analysts should have had an intensive training and should have appropriate qualifications.

Psychotherapy is not normally advisable for young children. This is because a young child can't really consent to the treat-ment, and may not understand the full implications of what is going on, and psychotherapy is normally only helpful when the client has consented to it and wants to take part. Children who have psychotherapy forced on them may resent it bitterly and it may actually be damaging to them.

Having said this, there is no doubt that some forms of therapy or counselling can be very beneficial for older children and teenagers. Many people do think that migraines can result from blocked emotions (see page 39). Sometimes migraines can be due to stresses and problems in the relationship between parents and child or to problems at school. Research has shown that migraines are more common in children where there has been divorce or other stresses in the family or when the child is unhappy at school, and some research has shown that psycho-therapy and counselling reduce the number and severity of migraines. Sometimes parents may need counselling from Relate or marriage guidance agencies if the strain of their child's illness is causing problems in their relationship, or if problems in their relationship are causing stresses for the child. In this way, the whole family can move forwards towards a positive future.

Chapter Six

As They Grow

THE PRESCHOOL YEARS: FROM BIRTH TO FIVE

Babies

It is now known that young children and babies do suffer from migraine. Often in a young child the attack is short-lived and may manifest more as abdominal pain and discomfort, often resolving with vomiting and sleep. Parents may not realize that their child is suffering from migraine until much later.

Case Study
'Henry had attacks of what seemed to be abdominal discomfort and vomiting when he was quite a small baby, at about six months. I just thought he had eaten some food which disagreed with him. For instance, for ages I didn't feed him avocado as he was ill and sicked up after eating one. It wasn't until much later that I realized that was probably coincidence. When he was two or three he started to say that his head hurt when he got these attacks, and the attacks usually ended with him being sick and then falling asleep, to wake up a few hours later much better.'

It is difficult to know what to do with a small baby who has migraine. As with older children, it can be important to make sure the child has a regular routine and gets enough sleep, although some parents think their babies' migraines may be linked to poor sleep patterns, about which parents actually have little control.

Some babies are very 'colicky' from birth – colic being a term which is applied to babies who cry a lot. The causes of colic are unknown. Originally it was thought to be stomach ache, but many doctors now think that it is more to do with an immaturity of the nervous system and poor sleep patterns. It seems that some babies have difficulty in relaxing into deep sleep – the slightest disturbance, internal or external, seems to wake them and they then cannot go back to sleep, no matter how tired they are, and cry in distress. It is possible that there is some connection between colic in a small baby and migraines; the baby may be oversensitive and the brain may be flooded with stimuli as happens in a migraine attack. Much more research needs to be done in this area.

It is very difficult to do anything about sleep patterns in a baby under three months of age. You can try keeping things very calm and boring at night – keeping the lights low when your baby wakes and feeds, only changing their nappy if necessary, and trying to return your baby straight to sleep – but often this doesn't work. 'White noise' cassettes which make sounds supposed to imitate those the baby would have heard in the womb are often very soothing. Some parents find having their baby in bed with them helps the whole family get a better night's sleep, others find they do not sleep well with their baby right beside them. There's no right or wrong about this, just do what suits you best.

From three to six months, you can help nudge your baby towards longer and better sleep. It is still probably necessary to feed your baby when he wakes, but otherwise try not to get caught up in walking up and down, going out for a drive, and certainly not playing with your child in the middle of the night. After six months, you can try 'sleep training'. This is probably what will be recommended if your baby's sleep patterns are so disrupted that you are referred to a sleep clinic. You will be told that when your baby wakes and cries you should go and reassure them, and then leave them to cry first for five minutes, then go back to reassure them and leave them for ten minutes, then fifteen, and so on. The first night will be hell, the second may be bad, but if you stick to this it almost always works by the third night.

Breastfeeding

Breastfeeding is the best and most natural way to feed your baby. Unfortunately, we live in a society where bottle-feeding is still the norm, and many mothers do not get the initial help and support they need to help them breastfeed their baby. Many mothers experience initial problems in getting their baby latched on, establishing a good milk supply and avoiding sore nipples. There are organizations which can help by putting you in touch with specially trained breastfeeding counsellors or supporters (see page 105).

Research has not shown any special link between breastfeeding and migraines, although breastfeeding has been shown to protect against allergic conditions such as asthma and eczema, and may protect against migraine which is allergic in origin. Research has shown that the breast milk helps line the infant's rather 'leaky' gut, helping to prevent foreign proteins from crossing the gut wall, and this may protect against allergic diseases. Further, breast milk contains many antibodies and immune factors which boost the young baby's immune system, and also attack bacteria, fungi and intestinal parasites. Breast-fed babies have lower rates of respiratory and gastrointestinal infections.

There may be other links between breastfeeding and migraines too. Most babies enter a state of profound relaxation after breastfeeding. This may be partly due to hormones produced by the mother being secreted in the milk. Mothers usually experience a sense of relaxation and well-being with the 'let-down' reflex in which the hormone oxytocin is released, the same hormone which makes the womb contract in labour and at orgasm. Breastfeeding can calm down a tense mother and fractious baby and may relieve headaches. Many mothers find that they do not experience migraines at all while breastfeeding.

Toddlers

The toddler stage – from about 18 months to three years – can be one of the most difficult and frustrating for parents and children alike. Toddlerhood is in a way like a mini adolescence, with the toddler striving for independence while at the same time still being emotionally and physically dependent on the parents and other carers. It is not surprising that because of this one of the most common words used by children at this stage is 'no'. Toddlers are also working out their relationships with children their own age at mother-and-toddler groups, playgroups and nurseries, or when small friends visit at home, and such encounters are often stressful, with a certain amount of jealousy, possessiveness and aggression being the norm. Many toddlers are also faced with the trauma of a new baby in the family at this difficult stage.

Dealing with tantrums

Getting tired and hungry leads many if not most toddlers to develop tantrums – the child with a tendency to migraine is likely to end up with a migraine attack too. The secret is to try to stop your child getting over-tired and to give him food before he is too hungry. The minute your child becomes whingy and irritable, try to find something quiet to do and give your child a healthy drink or snack. Take food with you in the car or on outings. When your child is enjoying himself it is easy to leave things too late and then suffer the consequences of tantrums, tears and a headache; it is better to leave before things get to this stage.

Tantrums can in fact be beneficial in releasing the frustration and emotions which the young child suffers, and it may be the child who does not have a tantrum but represses his feelings who is more likely to develop a migraine. Because of this, it is best to deal with tantrums gently and certainly not to punish your child for having one. The best treatment is quietly to ignore it and as soon as your child has calmed down a bit, to carry on as if nothing had happened. Don't slap, shout at, or manhandle your child and certainly don't get drawn into having a tantrum yourself.

A toddler with migraine probably won't be able to communicate the cause of his distress to you. A small child who is ill or in pain will usually appear to be irritable, clingy, and whining, which can cause the carer to become exasperated rather than sympathetic. Signs of pain in a child too young to talk can be the position of the body – often curled up, holding the painful part or clenching fists. Before the age of six many children do not really understand what 'pain' means, so to ask, 'does it hurt?' or 'Where is the pain?' can be meaningless to the child.

Sleep problems

Lack of sleep and disrupted sleep can make migraines more frequent and more intense. More than with a 'normal' child, you should try to keep him to a good bedtime routine and avoid late nights or over-exciting and stimulating games at bedtime. A bedtime snack or drink may also be beneficial.

If your toddler wakes frequently in the night, sleep training may again be beneficial. Once your child is out of a cot, it can be more difficult to ensure good sleep. Again, some parents find the solution is to have their child in bed with them so that everyone gets a good night's sleep. This doesn't work for everyone, however.

Case Study
'We tried having Ricky in bed with us, but he'd wake frequently, get very angry with us, and start hitting us or pulling our hair if we didn't respond to him. Then sometimes during the day he would be so tired that he'd go really pale, fall

asleep and sometimes he was sick. We realized later that this was migraine, but it wasn't clear at the time.

'Things got so bad that we went to the doctor and he referred us to the sleep clinic. They were very helpful. They pointed out that our whole family life was affected and that we were all bad-tempered with one another and miserable. The plan was simple. Ricky should sleep in his own bed. When he woke and came to join us, we were to quietly and calmly pick him up and put him back in bed. We weren't to talk, to shout, to do anything else. They told us that the first night we'd have to do this 50 times, the second night maybe 20, and the third night not at all.

'Actually I didn't believe them. This was confirmed by the first night, when I had to put him back in bed 147 times (I did keep count). The second night I only did it three times, and the third night, not at all.

'Life suddenly improved dramatically. Ricky started going to bed earlier and without a fuss. He was much more even-tempered and so was I. And he stopped getting his migraine attacks (these were diagnosed when he started getting them later at about the age of ten).'

Starting playgroup or nursery

Starting at pre-school playgroups or nurseries can be a stressful time and this may mean that your child gets more headaches or migraines in the short term. Migraine in young children is not widely understood and it is important to talk to the nursery nurses, playgroup leaders or teachers to tell them what the warning signs are and what to do if the child gets a migraine. You will probably want to go to the nursery or playgroup and collect your child at the earliest opportunity as few playgroups and not all nurseries have a quiet place for children to lie down.

If your child has dietary restrictions, it is important that the playgroup or nursery know about them. If your child attends nursery all day, it may be necessary for him to take a packed lunch, though he should eat this at the same table as the other children and perhaps eat 'safe' items from the main menu. (Lunchtime at nursery is very important for learning social skills and the children are often encouraged to serve themselves and one another.) This can cause problems on special occasions such as children's birthdays when sweets or cakes are often handed out. It can be an idea for the staff to keep some special 'safe' treats for your child for such occasions.

THE MIDDLE YEARS: FROM 5 TO 12

If your child suffers from migraine, then you will need to talk to the school and explain about the symptoms and what to do. You could ask the school if they will give your child paracetamol or other drugs; some schools are happy to do this while others are not.

If your child has frequent migraines, then missing school can be a problem. You can ask your child's teacher what your child would have been doing in class and try to make up some of the lost time at home. Sometimes your child will miss out on social events too – trips out of school and school journeys can all be disrupted by migraine.

It is best to let your child lead as normal a life as possible and not to stop him from taking part in all the activities that are on offer. In particular, you shouldn't stop your child going away on school journeys because they might get a migraine. It is important to talk to the teachers and tell them how best to manage a migraine. Often, a child will not get a migraine while away, but will have one when they 'come down' after arriving home.

As a child gets older, the pressures build up, and they can become particularly acute towards the end of primary school and parents and children often become anxious about which secondary school they will be going to and whether they will pass an interview or exam.

You can help your child through this difficult time by staying calm, and not discussing your anxieties with them. Praise your child – 'You are wonderful – I know you'll do well wherever you go' – and reassure them that whether they pass exams or not doesn't mean you will love them any more or any less. Don't force your child to work too hard – research has shown that doing homework in short bursts of half an hour or so is much more productive than spending hours on it. The brain can only absorb so much and too much studying is a sure recipe for headaches.

Sports

Taking part in vigorous sports can be a problem for children with migraine. Standing in the hot sun on a bright hard court or playing field can trigger a migraine, and violent exercise is another trigger. If low blood sugar triggers your child's migraines, as is frequently the case, ask if your child can be allowed to have a snack before or immediately after games.

THE TEENAGE YEARS: FROM 13 TO 18

As children enter adolescence, the stresses of puberty and secondary school cause an increase in the incidence of headaches in general and migraines in particular.

The teenage years are often difficult and stressful ones for young people today. Pressures at school to achieve are more severe than they have ever been, with traditional manual jobs disappearing and more and more careers dependent on educational qualifications, and more and more competition for jobs. In addition, young people are exposed to more choices, are bombarded with images of how they should be, what they should wear and things they should have. Social pastimes are often highly stimulating and tiring and many more teenagers will have late nights and hectic social calendars. In addition, more and more young people are exposed to alcohol and illegal drugs.

All these factors mean that more young people than ever are suffering from headaches and migraine. It is known that stress can affect migraine, as can sleep deprivation, alcohol and some other drugs. Dieting can also provoke migraines.

Some teenage activities seem almost certain to provoke migraines. Dancing in clubs with high noise levels and a smoky atmosphere, perhaps drinking alcoholic drinks and/or coffee and going to bed late to be followed by a long lie-in involves almost every kind of migraine trigger there is. Some people are robust enough to cope with this kind of treatment on a regular basis but others cannot.

You need to use common sense when dealing with a teenager who has recurrent headaches or migraine. Obviously your child can't miss out on all the socializing and experimenting which is part of the teenage years. Sometimes your child will have to stay up late at a party, and will just have to suffer the migraine which may then follow. You can help your child by supporting them and sympathizing, rather than saying, 'It's your fault for staying up till two am.'

You may also need to help your child make decisions about how to treat migraines. Once a child is over the age of 12 more treatment options are available and your child might like to use some of the new drugs which help prevent or abort migraine attacks (see page 51). Talk things over with your teenage child carefully. You may prefer the natural approach, but your son or daughter is becoming an independent person and may want to take another route. Or you can support them in choosing complementary therapies.

Menstrual migraines

For many girls, migraines start with the onset of their periods. There is no doubt that migraines are more common in girls after puberty than in boys, and two-thirds of adult (women) sufferers of migraine link their headaches to their menstrual cycle. It is known that hormonal changes can trigger migraine, and the contraceptive pill is known to aggravate migraine.

Migraine occurs at the same time as a period in about 15–30 per cent of women. More commonly, it starts with the premenstrual symptoms a few days before a period is due. Many of the symptoms of the migraine prodrome, tiredness, irritability, mood swings, also occur with the premenstrual syndrome.

Menstrual migraine was thought to be caused by a fall in progesterone levels but this is certainly not the whole picture. Migraines are in fact more likely to be provoked by a fall in oestrogen. Some research has shown that migraine sufferers seem to have a higher level of oestrogen and progesterone throughout their cycle.

Menstrual migraines are particularly difficult to treat and often do not respond to the usual drug treatments or even many alternative therapies. However, homeopathy, herbal medicine, nutritional therapy, naturopathy and bodywork are all great for balancing hormonal problems. One treatment which has been tried with some success is a skin patch which delivers an oestrogen, oestradiol, through the skin in the critical week before a period. This can be effective without changing the menstrual cycle.

The pill and migraine

Headache is one of the most frequently reported side-effects of the contraceptive pill. In one study, about 30 per cent of women suffering migraine said that their headaches became worse when taking the pill, and 10 per cent had not had headaches before but started them while taking the pill. One study found that the character of migraines could change, with women who had previously had migraines without aura being more likely to have migraines with aura when taking the pill.

A recent review of studies of the contraceptive pill did not find any difference in the different types and doses of contraceptive pill and the likelihood of their provoking migraine.

If your teenage daughter is sexually active then contraception is clearly important. If your daughter has migraines it may be worth considering alternative methods, and if your daughter starts migraines when on the pill it may be worth changing method. Although the pill is the most effective contraceptive, condoms are, of course, more effective in preventing sexually transmitted diseases, and it is important that changing to another method should not put your daughter at risk of an unwanted pregnancy.

De-stressing

One of the most important things for a teenager to do if they suffer from migraines is to reduce the stress in their lives. This is hard to do when all-important exams are looming and when children are going through the throes of first love, of friendships breaking up, and all the problems of adolescence. However, sometimes people who get migraines do burden themselves with more than they need to. You can help your child to realize that they don't always have to do everything.

Saying 'no'

Sometimes it is necessary to encourage your child to say no to extra work or activities, even though it can be hard for them. They don't have to be rude – saying 'I'd really love to, but I can't at the moment' will make it easier and mean they don't hurt the other person's feelings.

Don't set your child too high standards. It is much better for your child to feel a sense of achievement in reaching a more realistic goal than to feel they have failed.

If your child is under time pressure, help them to organize! Encourage them to prepare for the morning the evening before. Make sure they allow more time to get to appointments – and are not always running late. Don't rely on your and their memory – write things down. Don't allow homework or revision to pile up – encourage your child to get on with it sooner rather than later. Don't let your child leave projects or exam assignments till the last moment and then have to sit up half the night drinking coffee to keep going. Encourage them to learn how to pace themselves.

Conclusion

The Way Forward

By the time you have finished this book, you will see that there is much that can be done to help your child overcome their headaches and migraine. There is a wide variety of treatments, especially complementary ones, which will help relieve your child's headaches and/or migraine, make them less intense or long lasting and less frequent and possibly stop them altogether. They may have to try several treatments, but in the end they should find one that works for them. Remember, however, that they will need to allow enough time for a treatment to take effect. If your child embarks on one course of treatment, they should always give it a fair trial before switching to something else. There is every reason to believe that you will find a treatment which will help your child and provide significant relief.

Further, making changes in your family's and your child's lifestyle to remove stress, and improving their diet, can make an enormous difference. At first, making these changes may seem hard, especially if it means depriving your child of something they seem to want and which they are convinced everyone else is enjoying, such as frequent late nights, endless rounds of socializing and activities, and unhealthy foods. While your child is young, it is your parental duty to protect him, and once he is old enough to understand, you can explain that your child's headaches may be the price he is paying for his 'fun'. Your child may need and depend on you to say 'no' for him while he is too young and inexperienced to say it for himself. If you help your child at this stage, he will be able in time to take responsibility for his own health and his own body, and be able to manage his headaches and/or migraines or even learn to avoid them altogether.

Further Reading

MIGRAINE

Herzberg, Eileen, *The Natural Way: Migraine*, Element Books, Shaftesbury, 1994

Lewis, Jenny, *The Migraine Handbook*, with the Migraine Association (now Migraine Action), Vermilion, London, 1993

Rush, Ann, *Migraine – Understanding and Coping with Migraine*, Thorsons, London, 1996. Published in association with The Migraine Trust

Sacks, Oliver, *Migraine* (revised and expanded), Picador, London, 1995

ALTERNATIVE THERAPIES

Carter, Jill and Edwards, Alison, *The Elimination Diet Cookbook*, Element Books, Shaftesbury, 1997

The Rotation Diet Cookbook, Element Books, Shaftesbury, 1997

Castro, Miranda, *Homeopathic Guide: Mother and Baby*, Pan Books, London, 1992

Davies, Dr Stephen and Stewart, Dr Alan, *Nutritional Medicine*, Pan Books, London, 1987

Harvey, Clare and Cochrane, Amanda, *The Encyclopedia of Flower Remedies*, Thorsons, London, 1995

Hoffman, David, *The New Holistic Herbal*, Element Books, Shaftesbury, 1990

Lever, Dr Ruth, *Acupuncture for Everyone*, Penguin, London, 1987

Newleaf, G B, *Back to Balance, A Self-help Encyclopaedia of Eastern Holistic Remedies*, US and Japan Kodansha International Ltd, 1996

Price, Shirley and Price Parr, Penny, *Aromatherapy for Babies and Children*, Thorsons, London, 1996

Useful Addresses

Australia

Australian Natural Therapists Association
PO Box 308
Melrose Park
South Australia 5039
Tel: 8297 9533

Migraine Society of Australia
PO Box 2504
Kent Town
South Australia 5071

Canada

Canadian Holistic Medical Association
700 Bay Street
PO Box 101, Suite 604
Toronto
Ontario M5G 1Z6
Tel: 416 599 0447

The (Canadian) Migraine Foundation
120 Carlton Street
Suite 210
Toronto
Ontario M5A 4KA

New Zealand

New Zealand Natural Health Practitioners Accreditation Board
PO Box 37–491
Auckland
Tel: 09-625 9966

New Zealand Neurological Foundation
PO Box 68–402, Newton
Auckland
Tel: 09-379 8470

South Africa

South African Homeopaths, Chiropractors and Allied Professions
Board
PO Box 17055
0027 Gooenkloof
South Africa
2712 466 455

United Kingdom

Association of Reflexologists
27 Old Gloucester Street
London WC1N 3XX
Tel: 0990 673320

British Association for Counselling
1 Regent Place
Rugby
Warwickshire
CV21 2PJ
Tel: 01788 578328

British Homeopathic Association
27a Devonshire Street
London W1N 1RJ

British Society of Medical and Dental Hypnosis
42 Links Road
Ashstead
Surrey KT21 2 HJ
Tel: 01372 273522

Chiropractic Advancement Association (CAA)
PO Box 1492
Trowbridge
Wiltshire BA14 9YZ

Council for Acupuncture
179 Gloucester Place
London NW1 6DX
Tel: 0171 724 5756

Council for Complementary and Alternative Medicine
179 Gloucester Place
London NW1 6DX
0171 724 9103

Migraine Action
(formerly the British Migraine Association)
178a High Road
Byfleet
Surrey KT14 7ED

The Breastfeeding Network
PO Box 11126
Paisley PA28YB
Tel: 0870 900 8787

The Migraine Trust
45 Great Ormond Street
London WC1N 3HZ

Register of Chinese Herbal Medicine
21 Warbeck Road
London, W12 8NS
Tel; 0171 224 0803

Register of Traditional Chinese Medicine
19 Trinity Road
London N2 8JJ
Tel: 0181 883 8431

United States

American Association of Naturopathic Physicians
2800 East Madison Street
Suite 200
Seattle
Washington 98102
Tel: 206 323 7610

American Council for Headache Education (ACHE)
875 Kings Highway
Suite 200
West Deptford NJ 08096

American Holistic Medicine Association
4101 Lake Boone Trail Suite 201
Raleigh
North Carolina 27607
Tel: 919 787 5146

National Headache Federation
428 St James' Place 2nd floor
Chicago
Illinois 60614-2750

Index

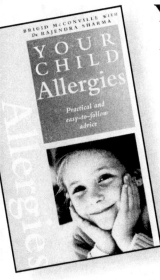
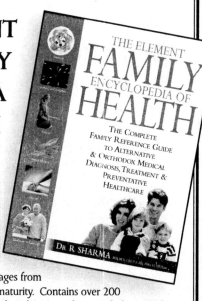
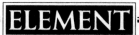

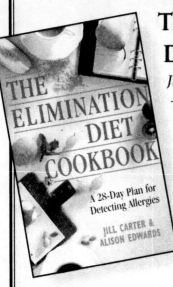
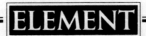

TO ORDER

UK: Please call the credit card order line on **0870 2413065** or fax your order to **01747 851394**.
For postal orders please send a cheque or postal order made payable to Element Books, together with your name and address
and the completed order form; (photocopies accepted) to: **Element Direct, Longmead, Shaftesbury, Dorset, SP7 8PL.**
Postage & packing free. *Please quote code YR2 on all orders*

US: Please call **1 800 788 6262** or Fax: **201 896 8569.** Please have your Visa, Mastercard or American Express ready.
You will be charged at the list price plus a shipping and handling fee and any applicable sales tax.

CANADA: Orders to: **Penguin Books Canada Ltd, c/o Canbook Distribution Center,**
1220 Nicholson Road, Newmarket, Ontario L3V 7V1.
Toll-Free Customer Service
Canada-wide Tel: **1 800 399 6858** Canada-wide Fax: **1 800 363 2665** Toronto line: **905 713 3852**

TITLE	ISBN	PRICE	QUANITY	TOTAL PRICE
			TOTAL	

All UK and European trade enquiries should be directed to
Penguin Books Ltd, Bath Road, Harmondsworth, West Drayton, Middlesex. UB7 0DA. Tel: 0181 8994036
For information on Element Books and how to order them outside the UK please contact your appropriate distributor.
(Prices correct at time of going to press, all books subject to availability)

AUSTRALIA
Penguin Books Australia Ltd
487 Maroondah Highway, PO Box 257, Ringwood, Victoria
3134, Australia
Tel: (3) 9871 2400, Fax: (3) 9870 9618

NEW ZEALAND
Penguin Books New Zealand Ltd
182-190 Wairau Road, Private Bag 102902,
North Shore Mail Centre, Auckland 10, New Zealand
Tel: (9) 415 4700, Fax: (9) 415 4704
or (customer services) 444 1470

SOUTH AFRICA
Penguin Books South Africa (Pty) Ltd
Private Bag X1, Park View, 2122 Johannesburg,
South Africa
Tel: (11) 482 1520, Fax: (11) 482 6669

CENTRAL & SOUTH AMERICA
Book Business International
Rue Dr Estdras Pacheco Ferreira 200, 04507 0 060
Vila Nova Conceicao, Sao Paulo SP, Brazil
Tel: (11) 884 2198, Fax: (11) 884 2198

PHILIPPINES
Penguin Putnam Inc.
375 Hudson Street, New York, NY 10014, USA
Tel: (212) 366 2000, Fax: (212) 366 2940

INDIA, SRI LANKA & BANGLADESH
Penguin Books India Pvt Ltd
11 Community Centre, Panchsheel Park,
New Delhi 110017, India
Tel: (11) 649 4401/649 4405, Fax: (11) 649 4402

PAKISTAN
Book Com
Main Chambers, 3 Temple Road, GPO Box 518,
Lahore, Pakistan
Tel: (42) 636 7275, Fax: (42) 636 1370

JAPAN
Penguin Books Japan Ltd
Kaneko Building, 2-3-25 Koraku, Bunkyo-ku,
Tokyo 112, Japan
Tel: (3) 3815 6840, Fax: (3) 3815 6841

SOUTH EAST ASIA/FAR EAST
Penguin Books Ltd
2nd Floor, Cornwall House, Taikoo Place,
979 King's Road, Quarry Bay, Hong Kong
Tel: (852) 2 856 6448, Fax: (852) 2 579 0119

SINGAPORE
STP Distributors Pte Ltd
Books Division, Pasir Panjang Districentre, Block 1,
No. 03-01, Pasir Panjang Road, Singapore 0511
Tel: 276 7626, Fax: 276 7119

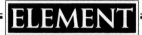